Use what was meant to take you out to lift others up.

Lisa G. Eley

LISA G. ELEY

Thirteen Geese in Flight

One Black Woman's Ascent into Mental Illness

Thirteen Geese in Flight: One Black Woman's Ascent into Mental Illness
by Lisa G. Eley

Unless otherwise indicated, the scripture versions cited in this book are the author's own paraphrase.

Edited by Tiffany M. Davis

ISBN: 978-0-9985-0180-2

First Edition

Printed in USA

In memory of my parents, James and Martha Eley,

who first taught me how to fly

and

to my goslings, Ashley and Crystal,

for being the reason why I still do.

Contents

Introduction: I Have Something to Tell You

The first time I spoke publicly about my mental illness, it wasn't planned. I was participating in a workshop when we took turns sharing trivia about ourselves. My group went last. Before I knew it, just when we were about to take our seats, I told the entire room of workshop participants how I'd spent time in the hospital under suicide watch.

Unrehearsed and delivered through voiceover cracks, fluctuations, and passionate anger--probably because I was trying very hard not to cry--I shared what had happened nearly two years earlier. What was divulged was hard to believe because what was said wasn't lining up with the Lisa they had known for some time. I always managed the business at hand very well and could be counted on to get any assignment done. Nothing appeared out of the ordinary to them, because I never let on anything was wrong. Had it not been for my impromptu confession, they still would not have known.

When my speech ended, I told them to do with it whatever they wanted. Then I sat. It was silent, way too quiet for an interactive workshop with a room full of people, who only a short time ago were laughing and joking about what some of us revealed about ourselves. From the looks on their faces they heard me, but were too stunned to digest it, a deer-caught-in-headlights moment. Some were crying, which made me feel so guilty for introducing sadness into what was supposed to be motivating discussions that I quickly countered with something I thought would make them feel better, even sealing it with a huge *Alice in Wonderland*, Cheshire Cat grin. It didn't work. The workshop moderator led me by the hand back to the front of the room. There, a standing ovation met me where the impromptu confession had ended.

What started out as journal therapy turned into *Thirteen Geese in Flight*, a testimony on how God lifted me from despair. The more I talk about it the easier it gets, where my tears no longer keep my spoken words company. Even now, people will look at me in disbelief until a hospital mugshot stirs a haunting visual of how far I've come.

Don't let the easygoing nature and smile you now see muddle your thinking into believing none of this ever happened. Many times I wish it hadn't and as long as God keeps my memory from waning, it is something I must live with for the rest of my life. If my going through it first means I've protected someone else from a wilderness few survive, then I've become a vessel God has used to help others avoid my fate.

"When we cast our bread upon the waters, we can presume that someone downstream whose face we may never see will benefit from our action, even as we enjoy the gifts sent to us from a donor upstream."
Maya Angelou

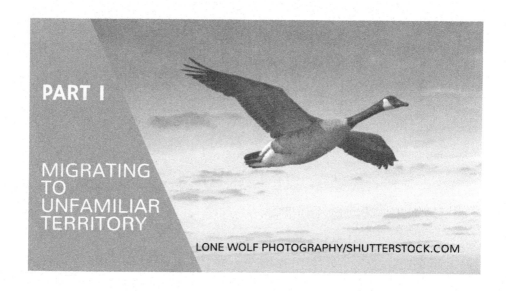

PART I

MIGRATING TO UNFAMILIAR TERRITORY

LONE WOLF PHOTOGRAPHY/SHUTTERSTOCK.COM

1 *Birds of a Feather*

I've always been intrigued whenever I'd see geese flying in V-formation. Ignoring their unanimously off-key, honking symphony, I would stop whatever I was doing just to watch this aerial show. It was never pretty at startup, but within moments the geese went from an unsynchronized conglomerate to achieving choreography worthy of an Olympic gold medal. How did they know to form a V, and which position to take in the formation flight? Was there a discussion at the resting pool, with lots of feathers drawn for their assigned flight positions? I once witnessed a goose so focused getting into position that he didn't notice the telephone pole cables in his path. Had it been a cartoon it would have been funny, but the poor creature hit the cables with such force that he was mercilessly whiplashed some distance back, leaving the cables rhythmically dancing long after I drove by, and after giving the rest of the flock a substantial head start.

Researchers say geese use the V for energy conservation during long flights and for visual acuity in tracking each other's positions in the formation. When a wounded goose falls from formation, others will join their fallen friend to help and protect it until flight can be resumed again. They will then catch up with their group, or head out with another formation.

This story is my journey into a place I would have never thought or imagined I'd ever find myself – bullied into depression and lost in suicidal thoughts. I dedicate this book to all of those wounded geese whose flights were interrupted through no fault of their own. May you take flight again, soaring higher and longer than ever before.

2 *First Steps of Faith*

I was stunned the first time my husband hit me. For better or for worse, I accepted his lie it would not happen again. After our second daughter was born, I wanted to believe the violence was behind him. I had just put the baby down to sleep for the night, having already dropped off my toddler at the home of my parents so they could take her to preschool the next morning. What had become the expected was now happening: my husband started in on me. Even when I walked away to avoid a confrontation, he kept the pursuit until he got want he wanted: a scuffle from me trying to prevent what he often took without consent.

People generally tend to steer clear of violence, unless they enjoy inflicting pain. It's a simple enough mindset and rational thinking. The fact that my husband frequently went out of his way to escalate a conflict--in spite of my avoidance--told me he liked abusing and violating me. Surrendering usually came quickly as not to wake up my older daughter, who often made her way to the melee with her dolly in tow and witnessed what was sure to scar any child. With her away for the night, he must have thought it was no-holds-barred, butt-kicking time.

On this late night, a few hours shy of the next day, we broke an all-time fighting record. Running more on adrenaline-charged fight than logical-thinking flight, the four-hour long rumble in the heat of the night destroyed a house that never

15

provided the warmth and comfort I had always dreamt my home would, as the safety and love of my parents' nest had done before I moved out. "OUCH," is what the walls must have said each time my husband would yank a phone from the wall to keep me from dialing 911 for help. If the walls could talk, they'd probably wish we'd be evicted so another family could appreciate its fine, brick frame and all that the home had to offer.

I did not want these walls to be my death trap. I thought if my baby girl had cried for her nightly feeding, then this would have possibly been enough to tame my husband's savagery and grant me a reprieve. But it wouldn't be so. She did something she hadn't done before: my daughter slept soundly all night. This added more fuel to the fire, which intensified my husband's desire to burglarize me even further. He didn't expect me to fight as long and hard as I did and, truth be told, neither did I.

Exhausted and battered, I convinced him to give me a drink of water and he agreed on one condition: I had to stay out of the kitchen where the knives were stored. Twice, during prior brawls, I had been able to cut him with a kitchen knife to thwart his attack.

Domestic violence awareness back then wasn't what it is today. Police never arrested my husband whenever they were called; they kept him at bay so I could grab a few bottles and diapers and leave the home, instead. I would move out with my babies and he would beg for my forgiveness with promises to do better. Peace was fleeting before he was at it again.

That night, when he left me alone in the living room to get the water, I took advantage of my lead and bolted upstairs to my baby's bedroom. In her closet were supplies I used for crafts, which included a pair of scissors with blades extending over five inches. I heard the refrigerator door slam and him running. It was dark as I reached inside her closet and pawed frantically in the place where the scissors last rested. I heard him land at the top of the stairs. That's when I felt the scissor handles and ran to meet him on the staircase.

He eyed the scissors and let out a dreadful noise--I'm glad to say--before he retreated. I sank to the floor, clutching the scissors, wondering how did I get here but, more importantly, how do I get out of this? Before I could finish my thoughts, I looked up to find my husband standing over me with the upright vacuum cleaner slung over his right shoulder like it was a Louisville Slugger and he was contemplating hitting a grand slam for the win. He told me if I didn't drop the scissors, he was going to drop me. Those scissors never left my hand and with that, I turned my back to brace myself and protect my head.

It was my first volatile relationship and I vowed it would be my last. It's been more than twenty years since I divorced him, never expecting him to divorce our children as well and launch my solo career rearing two girls. I told God if I survived the marriage, that I would spend my life devoted to Him. This was the beginning of my faith journey, and a life of tough breaks.

3 *Tribulations 'R Us, Inc.*

If there was a pageant for pain, I would have been crowned third, second, and first runner-ups, and Miss Hurt & Pain herself, all in the same contest. I made a second career of valleys below sea level and mountain peaks touching the sky. Obstacles was my college major, trials my minor. Had it been my job description, I would have earned Employee of the Year for a lifetime.

No sooner would I clear one hurdle when a more insurmountable one would appear. They seemed to come on cue, as soon as the slightest inkling of a breakthrough was detected. I tapped both of my shoulders with my fingertips and signaled God for a time out, a mercy break, strife no more. Tribulations 'R Us, Inc. was doing very well, thank you, and I was ready to sell the company.

I didn't expect to raise my daughters alone without a father's love and influence. After my beloved mother waited until we were alone to transition to heaven following a lengthy and painful illness, I didn't expect to lose my father a year later when his sport utility vehicle missed an exit ramp off the Baltimore Beltway and careened down an eighty-foot embankment, ending right-side up on Baltimore's Light Rail tracks. I didn't expect my big sister in Christ and beautiful friend Martina to succumb to cancer just months after celebrating her wedding. Nor did I expect a nagging back pain to lead to a major and risky operation. When my brother called to tell me our cousin Gregory had not been seen for some time, I didn't expect a detective to tell me that my darling angel here on earth had died in his home from natural causes. No one I knew would have wanted to walk an inch in the shoes of this poster child for some of life's misfortunes. Hardships were characteristically predictable in my life, and followed me like the musk from a skunk's offensive self-defense.

Have you ever focused so much on the short-term pain of a dentist's needle that it didn't register you were receiving medicine to numb the larger pain of a rotten tooth? Arthritis sufferers tell me this is how it was sometimes with cortisone shots. The initial shot was a doozy but the long-term comfort was worth it.

No matter what troubles came my way unexpectedly, I've come to expect God to sustain me for the long haul. If I could get beyond any present thorns in my flesh, I would be made all the better later after love, joy, peace, longsuffering, kindness, goodness, faithfulness, gentleness, and self-control (Galatians 5:22-23, NKJV) developed and strengthened my moral character. While my life at times may have felt like a point that went nowhere, a mock crystal stair made of eggshells, even the most painful experiences of my life were never pointless or unsalvageable. They made a good breeding ground for righteous living with eternal benefits.

In this you greatly rejoice, though now for a little while, if need be, you have been grieved by various trials, that the genuineness of your faith, being much more precious than gold that perishes, though it is tested by fire, may be found to praise, honor, and glory at the revelation of Jesus Christ, whom having not seen you love.

1 Peter 1:6-8 (NKJV)

4 *Launch Out Into the Deep*

My life, with all of its hardships, did have its occasional peaks of brightness. One of those bright spots came when I attended a Christian women's retreat to renew and rededicate my soul for faithful, fruitful, and Godly living. My very good friend, a recent widow, had treated me to a spiritual weekend getaway at the Gaylord National Resort in Maryland. Too blue for my blood, I'd visited the Gaylord only once before when my cousin and I reveled in a lavish, hour-long spa treatment, courtesy of her husband.

Convincing me to spend a weekend with sisters in Christ at a plush hotel was easy. Getting there was not. Always forgetting something, I had nearly completed the 40 miles to get there when I had to return home at the beginning of rush-hour traffic. Frustrated and inconvenienced on the second drive attempt, I heard a heart-stopping explosion and watched as a free-rolling blown tire from the camper trailer ahead aim right for my car. My heart felt like it had leaped from my body and smashed against the windshield, which was where this rubber death projectile was headed. I didn't brake or swerve, only watched in shock as this deer-sized tire lost steam and veered right, missing me and crash-landing without injuring anyone. The driver of the trailer pulled onto the shoulder, cars trailing me dodged the latest highway décor, and my heart didn't stop racing until I reached the hotel.

I almost called my friend to tell her I would miss the retreat. If it was this hard trying to get to the hotel--I thought to myself--then maybe I shouldn't go. Once I made it safely, the peace of God and the beauty of the Gaylord quickly calmed me down. I could already tell this retreat would be unlike any of the previous retreats I had attended. I felt a blessing was brewing that would change my life forever. While Satan may have tried to block me from reaching my destination, God made sure I would not miss my destiny.

Becoming a vessel God could use was the message for the women on the retreat. Once we exposed our wounds, exfoliated dead weight, and watered our cheeks, we launched out into the deep with workshops themed around the Sea of Galilee in Israel. Jesus walked from dry land and onto the sea, heading to the boat that was carrying his disciples. At first, the disciples thought Jesus was a ghost and were scared. Then Jesus spoke and told them not to be afraid. Peter, who was one of the disciples, stepped out of the boat and walked on the sea towards Jesus. But when the roaring wind spooked Peter, he started to sink and cried out for the Lord to help him. Jesus saved Peter but admonished him for his lack of faith. They both climbed into the boat, and the wind relaxed (Matthew 14: 22-33, NKJV).

Trusting God meant having faith. For a long time, I felt my personal and professional life needed something. Fear always held me back. Never the risk taker, I was always fine with the predictable and ordinary. However, the retreat seemed to confirm

22

it was time for a change, to go on a faith journey and get out of the usual. I was now willing to take that chance.

On the day I came home from the retreat, I received an unsolicited job offer from someone looking to fill a position. Word of mouth brought him to me. I didn't know much about him other than we had a mutual acquaintance in common. I was happy in my present job but now felt--in my heightened, spiritual, fresh-from-the-retreat state--a *rhema* word, confirming this was the change I needed, had been timely delivered to get me off the boat and into this new position. Peter received a similar confirmation when he walked, by faith, on the water after Jesus simply said to him, "Come." (Matthew 14: 28-29, NKJV)

The thought of learning new skills for work that was more aligned with my interests was compelling, but I had more reservations than you would expect from a person who should have been excited about a new job. Only God would know where this faith journey was headed. Unlike Peter--who almost drowned after he took his eyes off Jesus--I had to trust God completely to keep me afloat through strong winds, high waves, unrest, or anything else that could knock me off course and force me to sink. Out into the deep I sailed, not sure what to expect but sure I'd remain noble to my core values and primed to be a living sanctuary for God, as I've always strived to be.

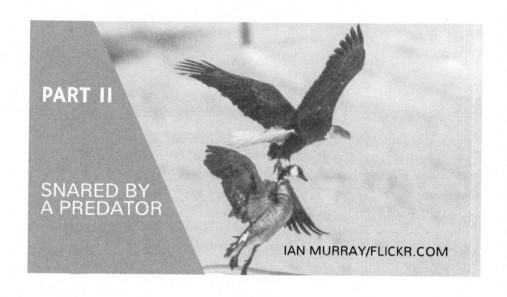

PART II

SNARED BY
A PREDATOR

IAN MURRAY/FLICKR.COM

5 *Saving Faith*

My decision to take that leap of faith and accept a job that made me unexplainably apprehensive came from inquiring of God for direction. There was nothing definitive spoken to my spirit telling me to walk away from the offer, so I went in with an open mind and heart even after I had heard questionable tales about this manager. I figured, if he had done all I was hearing, then why was he still working for the agency? He had some of the same staff for years. They had to be content, right? I believed then that I was taking the high road to hearsay with the forgiveness of a Christian. With limp red flags seemingly raised and uncertainty I couldn't validate, I made the lateral move to be trained and groomed under someone I perceived to be a respectable trailblazer.

It was apparent very early I had been duped, baited, and switched. The job was not like anything I was led to believe, or anything I had ever known. Management was eerily peculiar, with a dark and brutish philosophy. The man to whom I reported was shrouded in secrecy; transparency was an archrival to him. Neighboring offices smelled of life; workers were enjoying their jobs, each other, and their leaders. In our confinement under him, free thinking was not permitted and talking while working got you a condescending email.

While I understood there was some degree of supervisory separation and we were not equals, there was a vibe of subservience prevalent in our working death chamber. This supervisor and I were like oil and water, with opposing professional and personal values. Not only were we not on the same page, we weren't even in the same book and as far apart as two genres could be. He worked around the clock--weekends included--and tried to pass along an all-work, no-life balance onto me through subliminal messaging.

One example of this was his email policy. A heavy-handed emailer even when he was within talking distance, just about every email my manager sent was high priority. If I never saw another bold red exclamation point attached to an email, it would be too soon! You would have thought it was Outlook's default setting for the flurry of emails I'd get. For a job so physically laborious and work-packed, there was very little desk time for retrieving and reading them all, some of which were the size of a manuscript. Since my manager practically lived at work, he thought nothing of emailing me at four o'clock in the morning or eleven o'clock at night. He expected me to respond to his emails even when I was off the clock--weekends were no exception. I discovered why: knowing what my assignments were before clocking-in meant I could jump right into the workload each morning without "wasting time" on the emails.

I instantly rejected this notion, and probably not so subliminally, gave a neck roll and finger snap to boot. Law and disorder--working without pay, even if it was answering emails--

wasn't going to happen. This draft pick would not be a team player under such dictatorship and ill-thinking.

Shortly after starting my new position, my manager's sadism surfaced when he told me to come to work during Hurricane Sandy--even though the agency was closed, and the state of Maryland was in emergency status with all public transportation suspended. I had never seen such frightening weather in my life. Hurricanes were rare for our area. Schools, churches, government, and businesses were shut down because of the storm. The work I did day-to-day could have waited until the storm passed and it was safe to travel; there was only one of me. I was not going to risk my life to get to a job where I wasn't an essential employee and no one else was working. I didn't care if I had barely warmed my new office seat; I was done with this job and wanted out.

I asked for a transfer, but none could be given and I was stuck. My joy was depleted and my hopes went conspicuously missing with each passing day. This job was devoid of life and smelled of evil. The other workers were very nice and accepting of the stifling work conditions because without management support and references, they would not be able to advance their careers. It was the cruel nature of our field, and really unfair for some of the most brilliant and talented postdoctoral fellows there were; they were overqualified for many of the jobs they'd settled for. As minimum-wage workers, postdocs sacrificed more than most to build their careers.

Jobs were not as scarce for my type of position. I could get another job more readily, based on my own merits and strong work history, without needing a hand from management; biting the hand that fed me would not have me starving for long. My manager's power wasn't as great a hold over me as it was for the others. Once he knew I wanted to leave, he didn't make it easy for me to stay.

Having experienced unprecedented trials and circumstances, I tended to be very cautious in my decisions. I wanted an easy way out if things got too rough. Without warning, the boat I chose to board and launch out into the deep was now headed into the mother of all storms. I was being swept up in a black cloud where there would be no daylight ever again. I was going down with the ship.

6 *It Started With a Lie*

For everyone practicing evil hates the light and does not come to the light, lest his deeds should be exposed. But he who does the truth comes to the light, that his deeds may be clearly seen, that they have been done in God.

John 3:20-21 (NKJV)

It took residence in the farthest spot of my home workstation and was turned face down so it would be out of sight. My performance evaluation read like a personal pet peeve report of one-liners with objectivity, fairness, integrity, and reasonability all noticcably absent. With only three months' tenure under my manager's debauchery, my annual rating was "borderline failing." I could not believe this man, the filthy rotten scoundrel that he was, would start in on me with this asinine evaluation. My strong performance the prior nine months under a different supervisor, as well as from the past twenty-four years in public service, were apparently irrelevant. He must have been tooting his own horn while dancing to the beat of a crazy drum.

This was not okay. Down went the flag on the playing field. I challenged my evaluation for good reason: It was a lie.

How a long-term, senior manager in a leading federal agency could blatantly falsify my appraisal without remorse for its effects on my future employment, was beyond me. That was when

I knew for certain something was mentally wrong with this man. What was more astonishing was his gall and arrogance, to think I would roll over and accept this without a fight.

I could never have fathomed just how mean and unsavory a person could be, the lengths he would go, and lows to which he would stoop to mutilate my worth and obscure the truth. I had expected greater from a two-time Ivy League graduate, an anomaly who'd earned the highest and most prestigious dual-advanced degrees achievable. This painted picture alone would suggest supreme intelligence, upstanding morals, and common decency. Not so. This picture was worth few words, with *morale killer* and *evildoer* being my manager's best virtues.

The uneasiness I could not explain prior to starting the job came to light when I realized I worked for a narcissistic sociopath who relished tyranny, mastered revenge, and specialized in annihilation for sport. Granted, this was my nonclinical, unlicensed, and uncertified opinion, yet in hindsight I know was dead on. I didn't know what dysfunction was until then.

I lacked the privacy and time in a workday to place a confidential urgent email or phone call, seeking amnesty from my environment. My supervisor watched and timed every move I made. If, by chance, I was able to sneak and leave a message, it would be days or weeks before I received a response that offered no solution or promised no action.

I don't know what it's like to be a slave, work in a sweatshop, or be incarcerated but either, I surmised, was analogous to my job. Programmed to do as told and have no voice, I was a Stepford Worker in training to a wannabe tyrant. Then I did the unimaginable, my offense punishable by death: I had the nerve to shame my supervisor by going over his head to appeal my work performance.

To challenge a lie meant calling my boss out. I couldn't call him a bold-faced liar in person, but he was. The innuendo was the same, no matter how passive the wording in my facts-backed complaint - he lied. Because I told the truth and fought for what was right, I was rewarded with additional duties at a pace so brutal and inhumane I started to physically wither away. He had the power to do as he pleased.

Have you ever gone to a fast-food establishment during the lunch rush? The cashier takes your order while a runner fills your order. Occasionally the one filling the order disappears around the corner to give the cooks some grief, but returns to the front line to help with the rush. All hands were on deck because many hands were needed. In my situation I was essentially the cashier, runner, and cook all rolled into one, for a lunch rush that never ended, not even after the shift was over.

Going deep-sea diving without an air tank would be another way to describe my work situation. You surface as fast as you can to retrieve air. Before your lungs can recover and air has just barely found your mouth you are told to dive again, but deeper. You can't breathe, and you're woozy. Regardless, your boss does not want you to resurface until you have accomplished your assignment. Thinking he would appreciate your diligence, you make your way toward the surface on cramped legs and deflated lungs. Your mouth gets excited and opens prematurely, anticipating air coming to the rescue, but instead a smothering gush of water enters. You expect your boss to throw you a life preserver; instead, he only wants to know if you finished what he told you to do. When you admit that you have not, he calls you a failure and says your efforts were unacceptable. Your body concedes hopelessness and allows the sea to have its way. You drown, and your boss fills your position the next day.

The lunch rush and deep-sea diving scenarios were what it was like every day on the job. No sooner had I raced through one marathon day of work, then he would layer more tasks he knew were impossible to complete. It was my punishment for complaining about him.

The Israelites in the Old Testament suffered a similar fate. Pharaoh, the ruler of Egypt when Moses returned from a 40-year exile, would not release the Israelites from their labor. They worked like animals and were often abused. When the Israelites complained about their treatment, Pharaoh made their work more difficult. He demanded that the Israelites meet the same work quota by using fewer resources--Pharaoh refused to provide the straw the Israelites needed to make bricks (Exodus 5: 1-19, NKJV). My supervisor had a Pharaoh complex. He thought if I had the time to complain, then I must have needed more work to do.

A wolf in sheep's clothing, a demon in human skin, my manager hailed as the boss from hell, a crown he wore proudly. He suckled on the triple Ds of deceit, diabolicalness, and destruction. He was on a seek-and-kill mission to bully me non-stop until I didn't know who I was as a person or whose I was as a child of God. Do a web search of the Anti-Christ, and you just might find his picture. Any second, I expected his skin to shed and a forked tongue to flicker as he continued to squeeze the life out of me. If gratification was doing what felt good, then for him it was being cunning and callous. I would not be surprised at all if he got his rocks off from being demented. It all started with a lie his vanity never thought I'd contest.

7 *The Help That Wasn't*

I told the agency--and my boss--that I was under a doctor's care due to the stress from work. What I didn't mention was that my family doctor of fourteen years had placed me on antidepressants to help me cope with the job, and insomnia medication to help me sleep since I was highly anxious--a state of health my doctor had never seen me in before. When she was done examining me, she did something for the first time: she gave me a hug.

I was given an appointment with Ruth from Employee Relations. "How can I help you?" Ruth flatly asked, as she held the door to let me in. We sat down at the same time, and then I spilled out all of the complaints I had about the job. She maintained a strict business demeanor, even as she slid her box of tissues over to me. This was the first time I had cried at work.

For what it was worth, I also shared with Ruth many of the personal hardships I'd endured. I told her how I watched my mom's face contort and twitch, then relax right before she exhaled for the last time. I mentioned how I went to the Maryland State Police Barrack to retrieve my dad's bloodstained personal effects, after he had died in a one-vehicle crash. I finished by telling Ruth how--in the early years of my government career--I had to leave work during my lunch breaks to go to the food bank to feed my hungry family. I wanted Ruth to know that I was a professional survivor, and that I wasn't just whining over spilled milk. What I was dealing with at work was severely affecting my health, something my past tribulations had not done.

If Ruth really wanted to help me, she would have placed me in another position. A nationwide budget crisis and work politics prevented her from doing so. Instead, Ruth offered some rhetoric on perspectives, told me to work harder, and suggested I visit the ombudsman. Lastly, she gave me advice on looking for another job.

At the end of our meeting, Ruth looked at me and told me I would be all right. For some reason, I believed her. It must have been the parting look of sorrow I detected in her eyes (maybe she was human after all). It really didn't matter. I already knew before I left her office that nothing was going to happen to my supervisor.

Next, I sought the services of the Employee Assistance Program (EAP) and the Office of the Ombudsman. Both offices kept the same hours as my work shift. I needed permission from my supervisor to seek counseling during my work schedule. Permission was not granted and he would not join me at the ombudsman table. My boss believed that he was above coming to a conflict resolution meeting; he considered himself faultless. He told me my poor performance--and nothing else--was the reason for my problems at work.

For the few meetings I managed to schedule at the end of my shift, EAP would only provide stress-coping exercises, which did not amount to a hill of beans as long as my manager's mission was advanced stress infliction. The ombudsman wasn't much better. She made sickening passive offers, like asking if she should share my concerns with my manager. What good would re-telling the concerns he could have cared less about in the first place do, but elevate his mean-o-meter and diminish my life expectancy? I would have been better off sending a "bat signal" to the sky and awaiting the Caped Crusader himself to come to my rescue over what EAP and the ombudsman had to offer. Thanks for nothing!

Although they were both equally ineffective and useless for addressing my conflicts with my supervisor, the EAP counselor and the ombudsman were easier to talk to. Their demeanors were less rigid and guarded than Ruth's. I believe this was because their positions came with counseling credentials. They also had the ability to discern human behavior and body language because they were "psychological experts." My crying spells were just as intense with each of them as they were with Ruth. Either should have detected how high my stress and anxiety levels were. It was obvious I was affected by the events at work. This would have been the best time to nix confidentiality and alert upper management that they had a problem manager.

My survey responses following my final EAP session indicated my personal life was wonderful prior to the job, but my current work life was in extreme peril. For that, it was recommended that I have another meeting, which also resolved nothing. The only thing the meetings were good for was documenting my pleas for help. It's far-fetched, but I wish there had been a red panic button to alert the guardian angels of work/life equality and ethical treatment that one of their good and faithful workers was in trouble, and needed saving without a second to lose. Send in the cavalry!

As long as the stressor existed (he held a title and was my direct supervisor), prescribed medication wasn't going to help. The relaxation exercises from EAP were stupid, and it would only be a matter of time before the other shoe dropped.

My options were running out. Everywhere I turned for help failed. The next worst thing was a work detail. Details were temporary assignments--usually lasting no more than ninety days-- at another work site that required management's approval. The caveat of a detail was this: without assistance from the agency, you had to search for an unadvertised assignment to work. My manager denied my detail request--no surprise there.

Seeing that a work detail was only a temporary solution that would have required me to return to the job when the detail ended, it would have been far better placing me somewhere safe to work while there was an investigation to my complaints. At the conclusion of the investigation, an agreement could be made that would have satisfied both parties. This was wishful thinking.

I continued to reach out to Ruth after our initial meeting. She was my last hope for help. I started copying her on many of my emails from my boss so that she could read for herself the strain I was under. When she told me there was no need to copy her on all of the emails, I decided to call her so that she could hear the anguish and sense the desperation in my voice.

"He's giving me way too much work on purpose!"

"He's assigning what is expected of you for your grade and position."

"He won't let me take a day off to interview!"

"Schedule your interviews around your shift so you can get your work done."

"This is bullying!"

"No it's not."

Unfortunately, Ruth never grasped the magnitude of what the job was doing to me. The more we spoke, the more I realized I would never have her support. This was confirmed when I reached out to her (once again) with another complaint. "Perhaps, the position is more than you can handle," she rebuffed. This was crippling for someone who was declining fast, and it was the last time I contacted Ruth. Many more complaints would follow that were never spoken. They festered inside me, locked away. All was lost.

8 *Sinking Sand*

We were in the middle of a very large church celebration, paying homage to the man who had pastored tirelessly and led our church in an exemplary manner for the last 25 years. I had not slept or eaten in forty-eight hours. The nightmarish thoughts of the job stayed with me well into the weekends and would not go away. Moping around, attempting to do the Lord's work, I walked past a familiar sister who was bustling about with her hands full setting up for the affair. I greeted her with all the enthusiasm of a 2 a.m. infomercial on counting sheep. She asked how I was doing and I replied, "I'm dying." My stride never changed as I continued dragging this defeated temple of a body slowly along past her. It was enough for my sister to stop dead in her tracks and look at me like I was not half-crazy. Neither of us knew then that I was on my way to full-blown crazy.

Unscripted, with precision delivery and perfect timing, that's what I blurted out and couldn't retract. She heard correctly. Of all the things to say, that's what spewed from a spent soul. Things were not okay, I was not doing well, and I wasn't going to pretend to save face nor faith any longer. Still holding decorations for the finishing touch, my friend and sister in Christ brought her hands down, cocked her head to one side, and would not take her eyes off me. I insisted she continue with her tasks, promising to fill her in later when things were not as hectic. That's when she

41

made her way towards me and grabbed hold of me. Her loving hug and gentle prayer was all it took for me to let go and share what I had kept hidden for months. The job was robbing me of my sleep and appetite and, unbeknownst to me at that time, my mind.

I had suffered internally for so long that not even my family understood my mood change, nor had any idea I was in crisis from a job that was slowly killing me. The dishes would go for days before getting washed and I depended on delivery for meals because I gave up cooking. While one daughter was away at college, I stayed under my other daughter like a dog enjoying the sweet spot of a ray of sunshine streaming through a window. She probably thought we were having mother-daughter time when I entered her room each day after work and sprawled across her sister's bed. What I was doing was creating an artificial safety zone that gave me a sense of pseudo-comfort. I was no longer sinking; I had sunk. Bottomed out.

Self-encouragement took a back seat when I recognized this was a fight I couldn't win alone. It was time to enlist some Holy Ghost-filled spiritual warriors whom I trusted to help pray me through. My holy battalion would interlock arms in Ring-a-Round-the-Rosie fashion and not let me fall down. I was slipping but I held out hope, expecting and believing that God had loved me out of situations before, and He would do so again. I trusted Him with what dwindling sanity I had left because I was too afraid not to trust Him.

9 *When Praises Go Up*

Job hunting was a full-time occupation. With the sudden and intentional new overload of work assigned, plus the addition and imposition of warped, nonsensical, first-time deadlines keeping me toiling late nights and all weekends without compensation, my manager made sure I had no time to look for a new job. Discouraged beyond discouraged, I was desperate. Time was not on my side but I trusted God to deliver me into a place of purpose and calling by way of an exalted career shift. Until those prospective jobs surfaced, I redirected my agony by tending to the needs of others in my community.

Staying productive during a dry season I knew was temporary, but felt infinite, was the best way to mask the anguish in my spirit. I was trying to keep what little light remained from being completely extinguished. Doing good deeds for those in need had always reciprocated high feel-good dividends for me. There was no greater reward than being a blessing to someone else, the answer to a prayer. It's humbling to be used for good, whether a thank you followed or not.

The first time I volunteered to prepare and serve dinner at a residential treatment home for pediatric patients suffering from cancer, HIV infection, and other illnesses, I was surprised to see that none of the patients or their families were in down spirits. For an hour there was laughter, smiles, and fellowshipping that made you forget that a rare form of cancer was a dinner guest we did not want to honor for the evening. Families were thankful for the meal, and I got to witness children being children in spite of their circumstances.

That evening, our volunteer group visited the home to be of service to the patients and in return, they served me a scoop of gratitude for banishing my sadness briefly and allowing my appreciation for the little things to flourish. If I served God when all was well, then why not serve when all was not? His past goodness never depended on all being well and perfect in my life.

Exploring good works and encountering positive people delayed my shacking up with bitterness, even though I was still heavily flirting with sorrow. Praising God became a weak habit; I persisted, even when I didn't want to. Even in my solemn mood, my fear was I would become what I was dealing with if I stopped praising Him. Eventually I was going to have to pray for my enemy. By now, it was a real struggle not to want him dead.

10 *Deep in the Wilderness*

Lucas: "And Hansel said to Gretel, 'Let us drop these
breadcrumbs so that together we find our way home,
because losing our way would be the most cruel of things. '
This year, I lost my way."
One Tree Hill (Season 2, Ep.22)

The Brothers Grimm recorded the *Hansel and Gretel* fairy tale about a brother and sister abandoned in the forest by an evil stepmother when famine created a hopeless situation. The siblings ended up at the edible cottage of a wicked witch bent on devouring them to satisfy her lavish appetite. Believing all along God would not forsake them, the children outwitted their adversary and lived a life of overflow.

When I revisited this story, I had to get over the fact that someone in a maternal position would send two babies into the woods cold and hungry. I reminisced about my own beautiful mother who, over a Mother's Day weekend fifteen years prior, made the transition to eternal peace as I watched her take her last breath, ending years of suffering from complications related to diabetes and several strokes. I was so deep and lost in this wilderness that a trail of breadcrumbs--or even a neon-lit runway-- would have been of no use to me.

I raised my daughters to have purposeful, faith-filled lives but on this Mother's Day, I was grieving because my own faith was shrinking. An unusual amount of Mother's Day greeting cards found their way to my mailbox. I knew this was partly because I had been on the hearts and minds of some who were aware of my plight. Thank God, I didn't look like what I was going through because I was a holy mess in distress from a wilderness I wouldn't wish on anyone. I found myself fighting for my health, my sanity, my character, my peace, my joy, and my life!

Had God's number popped up on my Caller ID and I knew He was calling for a special assignment, I'd let the machine pick up. Never the spitfire and always the peacemaker, surely God had to know I was not cut out for this season's assignment. If He had intended for me to have a Jonah adventure and a great fish had heaved me out onto dry land (Jonah 1-2, NKJV), I would have been that person dousing myself with steak sauce and pleading for the fish to come back and swallow me again, rather than fulfilling this current mission. No one would have ever agreed to work under these circumstances, had they known beforehand what they were getting into. They'd make a fast exit, stage left, once they discovered the true gravity of the situation.

God, do you want me to die? I believed He did. I took a job in faith that was dire from the start, and I was ill prepared. I HATED going to work, being at work, and losing hope. And I was beginning to hate Him too, but with a lower case hate, because I had not heard from Him. Mother's Day was winding down.

Anxiety was aware of what Monday would bring, and it would be nothing good.

My Lord. Tomorrow, I face an enemy intent on hurting and destroying me. I've never seen this much evil and ugly so close, where acts of meanness are deliberate and continuous. Sunday's message was "Hope that Holds." Protect me, Lord, from his attacks and wickedness. I am no match for him as this is not my battle. The enemy has me believing I'm worthless, insignificant, inferior, unimportant, and unwanted. Yes, I am somebody's mother this Mother's Day but more important, I am your daughter Lord. Protect me, Father, and do not let me lose hope! Keep me close and deliver me whole, renewed, uplifted, and empowered into the plans you have for me. Only you know what's coming tomorrow, Lord. And I know whose I am and whose hope I'm holding onto. Amen.

11 *Staying Connected in the Valley*

My new routine each weekday was driving home through
tears and thanking God that one, I survived another day at work
and two, that my car avoided the same centuries-old Maryland oak
tree that kept beckoning me to drive through it. Community
commitments, contact with family and friends, and leisure
activities became things of the past as I went through withdrawal,
avoiding all things that used to make me happy. Friday nights had
me rejoicing because there would be no work the following
morning. Anxiety started to weigh on me by late Saturday.
Sunday morning church service gave me a quick fix that wore off
before I could even exit the church's parking lot and by Sunday
evening I was in full panic mode, anticipating Monday and the start
of another week of work hell. Come Monday morning, I wished I
didn't have to wake up. When I told friends this, they quickly
changed the subject.

Never before had my prayers and devotionals been so
intense. The soothing and encouraging tunes from my
contemporary and classic gospel music collection were now mute
to my spirit. God's presence was missing in action. It seemed I
had been disconnected from the Divine ISP hosting my spiritual
hotline and holy lifeline. Did I forget to pay the bill? I remember,
years ago, calling 911 to report a disturbance in the apartment
above mine. To my surprise, I reached a recording telling me no

one was available to take my call. Many hours later the police returned my call, wanting to know if all was okay. This was how it felt when I cried out for God to come to my rescue, but there was no answer. Months had gone by and I was still waiting for God to pick up.

I would come home from work and head straight to the sanctuary of my bedroom, where I would lie prostrate and beg God to do something. I'd heard countless testimonies where God delivered answers to prayers immediately, showing up right in the nick of time. I expected no less. I witnessed friends getting pink slips one week and a new job offer the next. That's the kind of delivery I wanted! *WHERE ARE YOU GOD, AND WHY AM I STILL HERE IN THIS SAME MISERABLE PLACE? I NEED YOU NOW, BUT I CAN'T FEEL YOU!*

Tears shed during this season surpassed all of the cumulative tears that I had cried my entire life. I was so mad at God, I started cursing Him out without using curse words, reminding Him of every single good deed I had done since I was born. Each spiritual tantrum ended the same way… with crickets chirping. God was tightlipped and the only noticeable sound came from the heaving of my own breaths from utter exhaustion. I was beyond done pleading my case to my Father and stopped caring.

12 *How Long?*

Trusting God in silence while hurting aloud, I had lost touch with reality. The only thing constant in my life was my battle with hopelessness. "It won't be long," I heard the voices say. *What won't be long?* I couldn't tell if these voices were in my head or if they were uttered from my mouth. I was slipping away, but to where?

Where was God's reassuring voice to break through the dense, pre-death air? At the very least, I should have heard the whispers of all His promises calming this storm and saying, *"Yet in all these things we are more than conquerors through Him who loved us."* (Romans 8:37, NKJV)

By now my bible had become a checkerboard of recently highlighted passages. Did I study these scriptures believing that sooner or later, good would win and evil would be defeated if I would just hold on and wait? *"For the vision is yet for an appointed time; But at the end it will speak, and it will not lie. Though it tarries, wait for it; Because it will surely come, It will not tarry."* (Habakkuk 2:3, NKJV) Or was I just doodling color highlights to kill time until I capsized and drowned, as in "The End" that God told the prophet Habakkuk was near? I made my own interpretive scripture, forcing it to blend with my gloomy mood over using it for its Living Word purpose. Because I hadn't heard back from God, I expected death to visit me at any moment.

The storm I was in had become too dangerous for a rescue attempt. I could have been told there was sunshine just around the horizon, ready to burst through the clouds, if I could tread water just a little while longer. The joy that was supposed to come in the morning must have gotten its days mixed up (Psalm 30:5, NKJV), perhaps because my nights never seemed to end.

I did not want to feel that all was lost, but despair followed me everywhere, all the time. It freebased my happiness, withheld my sleep, and anchored my soul in a pit of no return. I heard the voices again telling me, it won't be long.

For our light affliction, which is but for a moment, is working for us a far more exceeding and eternal weight of glory, while we do not look at the things which are seen, but at the things which are not seen. For the things which are seen are temporary, but the things which are not seen are eternal.
2 Corinthians 4:17-18 (NKJV)

13 *The Calm Before the Storm*

Had it been a boxing match, a knockout would have been imminent. The enemy's blows struck with expert precision. I surrendered before the referee could call the match. My last breaths on earth were coming to an end and I accepted the pilgrimage to death's door. *So this is how I'm going to die.* What other choice did I have? God had abandoned me. I'd been tormented for too long, for Him to just sit on the side, keep quiet, and let his daughter get beat up. I could get rid of the pain by either killing the source or killing myself. Either road--no matter how winding and chilling--led to peace, as far as I was concerned.

I began to forewarn family members and friends that if anything should happen to me, and I was unable to speak for myself, to look no further than my job. Premonition had me predicting my own death.

Management had hit me with everything--including the kitchen sink--above and below the belt, and was not going to let up until I was dead. The other workers felt really bad for me, woefully shaking their heads but saying nothing when they saw how I was being treated. "Stay strong," one whispered to me. "Good luck," whispered another on his last day before relocating to someplace better. Lucky him. He escaped the plantation, a word he used to describe the office. Never mind he wasn't even African American. If the agency would not listen to me in life, then perhaps they would pay attention to my death, since they would have been accessories to murder.

I began the tale of my journey with a harrowing account of domestic violence to set the stage for this moment in the story. I knew abuse firsthand because I'd lived it, and no one could tell me that my manager wasn't abusing me. Everything I endured at work would have been considered harassment and hazing outside of the workplace. Not liking my job took on a whole new meaning, when I confided in a friend as to why I thought there was violence in the workplace. It was because management bullies were driving some workers to violence.

Every time I wished my boss dead, I'd shake it off until those thoughts occurred so frequently they became dreams with different scenarios for action. Poisoning his coffee might only make him sick, not dead. A hunting knife in the right place would do. In the past, superficially cutting my ex-husband was intentional to stop his assault. Many times I wanted him to die in a car wreck, but never did I plot his murder. Now, the goal was my supervisor's instant death. What if I stabbed him in the wrong place and he fought back? Maybe I could pay some addicts to gang rape him, a death that wasn't physical.

I was not a gun owner. The background check that I knew I'd pass would have taken too long to obtain a gun legally. Maybe if I just went to certain places, I could "find" a gun. I knew people who owned guns, but would they let me borrow one? I decided to take full responsibility and act alone. No one else should suffer the legal consequences because I was preparing to kill the man who was trying to kill me.

Had my assassination plot turned real, I would have needed a gun for my own pain management. My conscience could have gotten the best of me, had I actually taken another life. So for the meantime, my boss avoided a date with death and received a grace period to live a little longer. I didn't know these were the thoughts of depression, or how long it would be before actions would speak louder than the figment of my imagination. This sounds disturbing, no doubt, but it's no more disturbing than work-induced mental illness brought on from a bully in a position of trust.

A wounded spirit said maybe I didn't have to kill him, only wound him enough to get him to stop what he was doing. A wounded spirit reasoned that my daughters were in a good place and months away from graduating from college, and would be okay losing me to incarceration for a justifiable vigilante-killing that would free me from psychiatric captivity. A wounded spirit didn't see that a human life would have been taken. A wounded spirit only wanted to stop the source of pain. To a hurting spirit, it was a matter of health or death.

My prayer requests had been consistent, but by now sounded like nothing more than a scratched vinyl record replaying the same miserable frame in the key of G minor. There was nothing minor about sadism. A select few knew who and what was burdening me, and were kind enough to check on me and offer encouragement. One was a church deacon who came to my home one particular evening to pray with me. My pint-sized dining room had become a makeshift church sanctuary and when the prayer ended, the Lord was present. I felt Him!

Pumped, I skipped the nightly sleep aids I had depended on for months and slept unassisted with only the high of the Holy Spirit, sleeping uninterrupted until it was time to wake up for work the next morning. That's when Hades was about to have the tantrum of all tantrums and the poop hit the fan. It got real...real quick.

14 *The Dream*

Police tape decorated my minivan as it sat in plain view,
just before the entryway to the baseball field. It was pitch black,
except for the lights from the police lamps. My rigor mortis-
stiffened form partially rested between the front and middle seats,
and was the fixation of the flash bulbs from the police cameras.
Living in a city ranked as one of the top twenty-five places to live,
we weren't crime free but finding a dead body was highly unusual.
I chose this popular residential park to end my life, to spare my
daughter from finding my deceased corpse in the house.

I sat straight up in bed from this surreal dream, just before
the alarm clock was about to beep. I'd had fleeting thoughts of
suicide before but never pictured the end result. By this time, I had
yet to make the pleasure of acquaintance with clinical depression.
There had not been an official diagnosis. All I knew was I'd been
very sad for a long time, and just saw my dead body in a dream.

Dammit! Time to get ready for work and more hell,
picking up where yesterday's torture left off. It wasn't quite
daybreak when my daughter yelled from downstairs that she was
leaving for her job. I didn't know she was scheduled to work that
morning but I told her goodbye, and to have a great day. The front
door closed and the depressed mind--which was still a stranger to
me--told me now was a good time to do it. Depression coaxed me
to kill myself while no one else was around. No sooner had that

thought came, when another thought told me to get to the hospital. Two opposing thoughts--die or live--were overlapping and racing against time.

It was a showdown at high noon, only it was just about six in the morning. I stared down my stash of prescription drugs and they stared right back, forcing the biggest game of "Chicken" I had ever played in my life. My fingers were itching to uncap the bottle of pills. I trembled so hard that I kept dropping my pen; therefore, I decided not to write a suicide note. The method of choice for ending my life was within arm's reach. The phone to call for help was a mile away. The blurred, fine line between the two became taut long enough for me to decipher lucidity from lunacy. I left an emergency message for my doctor, phoned a friend, and drove myself to the hospital. No family, no friends, only me.

It took three miles to get to the nearest emergency room (ER) on a mind that was not sound. Three employees were having a light-hearted conversation when I approached the admissions counter. When they saw me, they stopped and dispersed, except for one. The woman seated behind the glass partition asked if she could help me. Even though I was the only one in line, I leaned over and whispered something barely understandable to myself. She asked me to repeat what I'd said as we both leaned in closer. "I'm having thoughts of hurting myself," I whispered a little louder.

She took some rudimentary information down and without having to take a seat in the waiting room, I was buzzed through the security doors and met by a nurse. I answered every question she asked, including my method of choice for taking my own life. Inside my purse were two prescription medications I'd hastily grabbed before leaving for the ER. These were the same medications that my primary doctor had prescribed to me three months earlier. I hadn't been referred for psychiatric help then because events had yet to reach the boiling point that brought me into the hospital this day.

The ER routine was not new to me, having been a repeat offender for a bout of vertigo, among other things. Leave a sample, get undressed, lie on the gurney, and a doctor will be in soon. The one difference today was that I had a babysitter to thwart any plans I might have had to harm myself. She even guarded my purse and kept it out of my reach, although I was permitted to have my cell phone for the moment.

The first person to enter my room was an ER nurse, who asked me what was going on. I couldn't stop sobbing but told her the same as I'd told the admissions clerk, only now adding why I wanted to hurt myself.

My supervisor was bullying me nonstop, working me to death in retaliation for complaining about him. This had been going on for months, funneling the perfect storm that had delivered me to the ER that day. He had gotten into my head and had taken my mind on a joyride, playing a dangerous game of id, ego, and superego tampering. Like a volcano, there had been numerous warning signs leading to the eruption. But like a Maryland earthquake, my psychotic episode came unexpectedly.

The nurse was very compassionate and told me I did the right thing in coming to the hospital. I shed tears of relief and gave much thanks: I finally had some hope that someone was listening, and believed me.

A jarring thought jolted me back to the present. It was a few hours past my report time for work. In spite of my state of mind and current condition, and even before I had a chance to notify family of my crisis, my thoughts turned to the job because my manager would sure enough charge me with AWOL, an unauthorized leave of absence from work. He had done so before when I took a day off for a job interview he knew about. The thought of even communicating with him had me fretful. I asked the nurse to please call him and let him know I would be absent. I didn't know his number, so I just gave her his name and the agency. Bless her heart, she didn't hesitate to do so. She located my manager and took care of it. The job was covered; I had an excused absence.

When the ER physician entered and sat at the foot of my hospital bed, he too asked what happened. I cried my way through another round of describing my punishing misery of a hell pit created from abuse and a hostile work climate. After finishing my tale of horror, I looked up through waterlogged vision at this man of medicine and was met with the kindest eyes I'd ever seen. They were blue-gray beautiful, outlined in mist as if he wanted to cry along with me. That was something I couldn't quite comprehend because, by the nature of his profession, he was conditioned to handle the grimmest of trauma and remain detached. His role for that morning was nothing more than to patch me up and move on to the next patient. As long as I live and have a mind to remember, I will never forget the look of care and sorrow he had on his face. In an instant, he represented everything that management was not.

We connected. One look at me, and the doctor got it. He felt my pain right away, something I couldn't get my agency to do. Extrasensory perception (ESP) had nothing to do with it. Anyone with sight and a heart could tell I had been traumatized. *Damn the agency!* Maybe this damsel in distress saw her knight in shining scrubs coming to her rescue, when all seemed hopeless and lost. Everything about him said I would feel safe and not have to feel afraid anymore.

He, too, told me I did the right thing by coming in, and arrangements were made for me to meet with a crisis counselor. Thank God for compassionate people, angels here on earth, and another glimpse of hope.

While waiting for the counselor to come, I contacted family and friends before my cell phone was confiscated. I sent a text message to my daughter, telling her I was being admitted to the hospital to finally get the help I needed and for her not to worry. Later, she told me that she broke down on the job as soon as she read the text, so her supervisor excused her for the day. Next, I called my brother and told him why I was in the hospital, and that it was all due to the job. He pleaded with me to hang in there and I cried all the more, because I had been trying to do just that for months. The last few texts and emails went out to close friends and family, letting them know I was having what I thought was a nervous breakdown, and was being admitted to the hospital. It was barely nine o'clock in the morning but, as I was told later on, they saw my message but couldn't believe what they were reading.

It was a surprise to me and everyone else because we did not understand the effects of bullying on mental health, and why my job sat idly by and let me go to waste. It turned out that for all the complaints I'd lodged against my supervisor, the agency said I wasn't being bullied. Chicken Little had more believers thinking the sky was falling, than I had convincing the agency management was abusive. Depending on which version you read, Chicken Little perished after being lured to the fox's den before she had a chance to tell the king the sky was falling. Unlike Chicken Little, I didn't perish before getting a chance to tell the higher-ups what was happening to me. Having been in the bully's den for ten months, I nearly perished after they already knew. For the foreseeable future, my new job description would be recovering from a bully.

15 *The Reality*

I don't remember if she spoke and introduced herself, but I do know she annoyed me right off the bat. The social worker--the superhero for the disenfranchised--took a seat beside my bed and sat her coffee down on the floor, beside her chair. She angled her clipboard toward my head like she was preparing for an inspection, ready to eagerly tick off deficiencies. Who stops for a cup of coffee before seeing a patient in crisis? Sensing her gaze on the side of my face and with neither one of us having anything to say, I became fascinated with the ceiling architecture.

Why is she staring at me? "Are you waiting on me to say something?" I asked at last. I refused to break my ceiling trance.

"Yes," was all she said, before she shifted forward in her chair.

I sighed, continued to address the ceiling, then cried on cue through the same account I had given earlier to the triage nurse, the ER nurse, and the ER doctor.

From the corner of my eye, I saw her pen stop moving and her grip on the clipboard relax. Curiosity made me turn my head to see her reaction. If a doctor was nearly swayed to tears by my story, then this was all in a day's work for this woman. I read nothing; I got nothing. The only thing she was moved to do when I was done talking was reach down for another sip of her coffee. "I think you should be admitted to a psychiatric hospital."

A psycha-whoee? Did I just hear correctly? Just like that, I stopped crying in midstream to grasp what she had just said.

"Isn't this something that the doctor and crisis counselor should decide and discuss?" I asked.

"I am the crisis counselor," she replied, matter-of-factly.

Wow! What a surprise. Ms. One Shade of Dull delivered this news without batting an eye. *This is who you send to intercept a suicide?*

I didn't care if I wasn't well; she'd just earned a bona fide reading. "Everyone I've met at this hospital, to this point, has been warm and sympathetic but you. You seem cold and distant. Why haven't you told me I did the right thing by coming here? Everyone else did! You don't even care!" Her patronizing echo was dryer than the Sahara Desert and sounded like a robot recording: "I-care-a-bout-you-and-you-did-the-right-thing-by-com-ing-in."

While I was still trying to analyze her "gift" for crisis management, she told me that becoming a psychiatric inpatient would protect me from myself. I'd never had a VIP (Vanish Into the Psychotic) invitation before. It was far too overwhelming. I should have had some moral support from someone who could help me mull over this decision. I had two burning questions. First, would I be safe and second, could I leave when I was ready?

All I knew about psychiatric hospitals was what I'd seen in the movies, where someone always ended up dead. *One Flew Over the Cuckoo's Nest* was my sole source on all matters mental, I told her, which was enough to draw a hearty laugh from the crisis manager. I even gave a slight chuckle, which was an amazing feat under the circumstances. After she explained what I could expect as a psychiatric resident, my breathing returned to normal and I agreed to be admitted.

Thoughts of my daughters came to mind as I wondered if they would take me to some long-distance, aloof place off the beaten path. I asked where this place was and the crisis manager told me it was right behind the main hospital. Wow, part two! An ambulance wasn't going to whisk my restrained body away to the abyss. There would be no straitjacket and my transportation would be a wheelchair. As an accident-prone, frequent visitor, card-carrying member of this hospital's outpatient surgery services, I had no clue they offered psychiatric care on site.

The last thing I expected was becoming a psychiatric patient before the day was over. The plan was to shut down the pain, even if it meant shutting down me. I was ready to leave this earth but for now, I was relieved because I had been spared from death. Thinking a few days rest should do me good, I was ready to begin this new journey. It was obvious I knew nothing about the world of mental health care management to come. Covered in blankets with my belongings in a brown paper bag across my lap, I was given a security escort while a nurse wheeled me to the psychiatric wing. No pun intended, but it was a bumpy ride from the start.

The path we took to my new home was not conducive to wheelchairs. It felt like roller skating on top of gravel. Outside of my fanny being sore, the view from the windows along the way showcased an enchanting, immaculately manicured lawn enclosure dressed in flowers. There were perfectly decorated walking trails and exquisitely crafted wrought-iron benches. It had been early morning when I arrived at the ER, but now the sun was in rare form and saying hello, and inviting me to come out and play. I could see myself leaning my back up against one of those trees with a book in my lap and communing with God, giving thanks for the gentle breeze massaging my soul. I would slide all the way down the tree and lie flat on my back, making a grass angel with my arms and legs, only lifting my head up occasionally to make a dandelion wish, then blow.

I thought my outdoor playpen was waiting for me as the guard held the door for my wheelchair to cross the threshold. What I hadn't noticed in my euphoria was a very tall iron fence moving closer and closer. Even from afar, I could tell what waited on the other side of the fence was dreadful. My assumption was correct, as we moved along. The grass was less kempt, the flowers few, and the rattling of the security guard's keys guided my attention to the padlock he was about to open. I recoiled at the sound of the gate slamming closed behind us. In a few yards, I had traveled from calmness to calamity.

I was deposited onto a ward in a psychiatric hospital and told to have a seat until a nurse could check me in and over. This was a co-ed unit, with some patients walking around in only their gowns. Wow, part three! My tears had already gotten a head start. Within a few minutes one of the gown-clad patients came over, extended his hand, and introduced himself. A mocha caramel brotha I would have considered fine, if our age difference was a single digit and we both weren't mental patients. *Excuse me? Did I ask to make your acquaintance?* Not looking at him, I feebly answered "I'm Lisa," before I reached up blindly. I hoped it was his hand I had shook from my seated position. It was!

Right then, another patient was having a tirade at the nurses' station. While the nurses calmly engaged her to reach a solution that would make the patient less animated, the other patients paid her no nevermind and continued with their conversations, moving about like it was nothing. The only one staring at this exchange was me. Fear immediately seeped down into my belly, having been on the ward for less than five minutes. I wasn't like any these patients, wasn't feeling any of this, and resented being there. I was a voluntary admission; now I was ready to voluntarily leave.

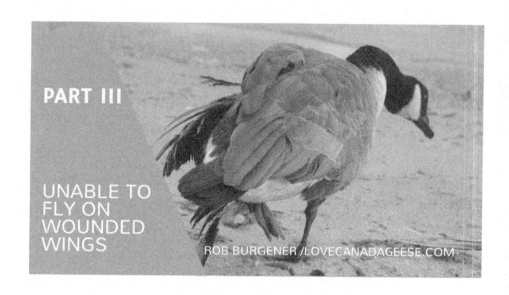

PART III

UNABLE TO
FLY ON
WOUNDED
WINGS

ROB BURGENER /LOVECANADAGEESE.COM

16 *Officially Doing Time*

I could have lost my mind, but for Jesus. How many testimonies and gospel melodies spoke on the mind that almost got away? Depression deafened God's voice and invaded my spirit. My mind was the one that got away. It was gone and under shared control of both good and bad consciences. I found myself in treatment to help recoup my lost mind, requiring a lengthy stay in a halfway house, the number of days to be determined.

I learned fast what it meant to be an inpatient on a behavioral health care unit. Two nurses had me disrobe and reveal every mark, blemish, and scar I ever had, no matter the location. My belongings were inventoried and taken away, my shoestrings were removed, and I had to surrender my cell phone. Staff became TSA screening agents. Anything visitors brought to the unit had to be scanned and thoroughly inspected. When my cousin brought over some head wraps during one of her visits, we found out they posed as asphyxiation hazards--much like shoestrings--and had to go back. Tough luck if you were a female and a male handled your unmentionables. Bashfulness had no place on a psych ward.

The euphoric garden image that made me believe my mind could run away and escape had only teased me, and been replaced with windows where you could see neither in nor out. On any given day it could be sunny or rainy; you'd never know the difference. No birds, butterflies, flowers, or even grass. This was what it must have felt like to be an inmate in a maximum security prison.

The one door leading in and out of the unit remained locked and my first visitor through the portal to nowhere was my daughter. It was not visiting hours yet, but she had been granted special permission to see me briefly since I had just been admitted and was alone. All she knew was that I was fine when she left for work and a few hours later, I was in a psychiatric facility via an emergency room stop. During her visit, she told me she started crying when she arrived at the ER and a nurse took her aside to deliver what my daughter thought would be the news no one wanted to hear: your loved one was gone. Instead, she was told I had been admitted for psychiatric treatment. I looked at a younger reflection of myself and wondered if she understood all that was happening; I sure didn't. For the way these young people stay on their smart phones and gadgets, I suspected had I actually killed myself, I would have turned to dust before my daughter realized she hadn't seen me in a while. I asked her for my bible and a change of clothes when she came back to visit.

By now, word had reached other family members and close friends. They knew I was having problems on the job but my God, they had no idea it was bad enough to come to this. They encouraged me to focus on getting better and wondered what kind of person I had been working for to cause such a thing.

For the most part, I got to lie in bed undisturbed the first day, except for when the staff checked on us every half hour to make sure we were all accounted for and among the living. It seemed suicide attempts did not stop once you were admitted to the hospital. Staff wore first name-only badges with their last names redacted. My meals were delivered to the unit and I ate in solitude, while acclimating to my real-life playpen. The ward was the length of two mid-size grocery store aisles set end to end. The chairs were so heavy, it was an effort just to scoot myself up to the table to eat. They were designed this way to deter lifting and throwing.

The common room was lit with cheerful, childlike artistry covering the walls, no doubt the masterpieces of prior patients. There was one television, one outdated computer, and enough board games to keep the castaways on *Gilligan's Island* busy, never to be rescued. Pencils were shorter than a child's finger, another anti-weapon caution, and too small for even an old-fashioned grade school compass.

Shower shoes, magazines, and cash for the vending machine were all I wanted for now. Thanks to my good friend (the one whom I called at the onset of my crisis), she delivered them to me before the night was over. The nurse taking my vitals for the evening asked where I worked, and I told her. She went on and on about how good my job must be until I had to shut her down and tell her my job was the reason I was there.

For the first time in a long while, I was actually looking forward to waking up and facing a new day. The night brought the best rest I'd had in a year because I knew when I awoke the next morning, I'd be safe from harm. For now, my desire to die had been delayed.

17 *Day Two*

It was a little after six in the morning when I awoke. No one else was up and the nurse told me it was too early to shower. Thoughts returned to the job while I retreated to the peace and quiet of my room. My roommate was still asleep, wrapped in her blanket like an insect in a cocoon, ready to be sprung. I had startled her the day before when she barged through the door and stopped dead in her tracks; she didn't expect to find a collapsed and dejected life form sitting on the other bed. I spoke first, Princess said hi back, and then she kept it moving. She was younger than my daughters, so we had nothing remotely in common.

I got back in bed and read until the only clock on the ward, halfway down the hall, gave us all permission to get up. I flipped opened my devotional book and arrived at *"Behold, I will do a new thing; now it shall spring forth; shall ye not know it? I will even make a way in the wilderness, and rivers in the desert."* (Isaiah 43:19, KJV) Rational thinking and many prayers had me believing my escape route from management's clutches involved God opening a door to a new job, not an asylum. You've got to appreciate God's timing, or His sense of humor. How grateful I was that my ways were not His ways (Isaiah 55:8-9, NKJV).

Already my first few days as a person being treated for mental illness were far better than the past year spent with the enemy. When I gave up and let go, God interceded and took control of the reins. He had not forgotten me; He knew what He was doing. I thought that a job change would have fixed everything. Now I realized that my mind was not in the best place to start a new job; I would have carried over too much baggage from being wounded and vulnerable. I had to first get well before I could work anywhere else again.

No longer a newbie, day two afforded me the luxury of taking a field trip to the cafeteria with the other patients and a staff escort. It felt like I was back in kindergarten at Baltimore City Public School #224, with a teacher leading us to the school library for a reading of *The Five Chinese Brothers*. The job had stifled my appetite to the point where I forgot what it was like to sit still and enjoy a meal. Eggs, sausage, potatoes, raisin bread, coffee, and apple juice from the hospital's kitchen made for a divine array of perfectly blended nourishment, with all the imaginative aroma of a French café. Sipping and savoring collided with the cheerful breakfast rush chatter and obvious daylight from my first unoccluded window in nearly twenty-four hours. Seeing sunlight awakened my atrophic soul from a spiritless slumber because even while I was becoming reacquainted with the pleasures of smell and taste, sadness was still the flavor of each day.

The breakfast conversations of my fellow ward mates brought me out of my deep thoughts. Someone shared an EMT (emergency medical technician) story of why a car passenger should never stick his foot out from a moving car's window and the answer was appalling. *If this was the topic of choice for a breakfast conversation, then maybe you belong in here,* I thought. I didn't judge his next comment because I believed him when he said anyone could be driven to kill, if pushed. I was bothered more by the equal opportunity, freestyle cursing intermixed in the discussions, than by his latest assertion. It was enough for me to tell a female staff member that the language made me uncomfortable. Being offended by the profanity should have been the least of my concerns. As with everything else, from hazard-proof furniture and windows without a view, I made a quick adjustment to the language.

Whether we wanted to or not, we were supposed to participate in the group sessions. Asking an emotionally unraveled introvert--one day removed from suicidal ideation--to open up to strangers was not the brightest idea to me. In fact, I'd say it was absurd. Each morning began with an assessment exercise asking us to rate how we felt on a scale from one to ten. Halfway down the sheet was the question that always followed you once you've been identified with a mood disorder: "Do you feel like harming yourself or others?"

Four was my rating this day. I was sad to be in a behavior health facility, mad at my supervisor for causing my mental breakdown, and very worried I would have to return to that ratchet place once I had been declared fit and well.

The unit's social worker communicated with the agency on my behalf, at my request. My worry turned proactive after the

75

social worker reported that management asked how long would I be in the hospital. My mind heard, "When is she coming back so I can finish her off?" That's when I wrote a suicide note and gave it to a nurse. I hated management and was angry the agency did nothing. I didn't ask for, or deserve, this interruption to my life. It wasn't enough that my boss sabotaged my career and had tried to force my resignation; he tried to make certain that I would die. That's what killers do. He knew *How to Get Away with Murder*, sat on top of a pedestal and presumed *Empire*, but only brought shame and *Scandal* to a field and agency known for long-standing, credible public service. Managers are becoming the new terrorists. Boom!

I asked for a copy of my suicide note more than once, and each time was told I'd get one. Pun intended, now I know that they had psyched me out and had no intention of accommodating my request.

Soon, calls from my loved ones inundated the hospital's switchboard. Their expressions of concern and support helped lift my mood. Understandably, there were some who wanted management's head on a chopping block, including me. Had I enjoyed such vigilante justice, I would have been no better than him. Others dropped his name on some prayer warriors to, in the words of one, "get him the hell off" me. A few days in the hospital and I was already breaking one of the Ten Commandments: I met the man I considered to be my second God, the psychiatrist charged with taking care of my mind.

I wandered into group sessions, prescription casting calls, spot checks, and psychiatrists to go – the Healing Games, where the objective was for everyone to survive, not perish. I had taken another step on the road to recovery. Day two in the hospital was in the books.

18 *Day Three*

"Code White! Code White! Code White!" Lights started flashing from the ceiling and the intercom announcer would not shut up. The nurses gathered us in haste and said we had to go...now!

Code what? Where are we going? Being secluded without a window view leaves you oblivious to pending natural disasters. A tornado came to visit, but I wasn't home to answer. Of all the places to be for a tornado to touch down, my current residence and limited place for refuge made me nervous.

Herded like cattle down a narrow basement passageway, we left the confines of our unit and linked up with patients I hadn't seen before. We had been housed on different wards--depending on our illnesses--and would have never crossed paths in the hospital. Packed like sardines, we merged and lined the oatmeal-colored walls of what could have been a bunker in past wars, and waited the weather out. Claustrophobia and anxiety overtook some of the other retreating, tunnel dwelling inhabitants; it must have been too scary and crowded for these patients, whom staff had to calm down. The wall was my support until it, too, grew weary. I eased down onto crouched knees, where I buried my head in a book. I only pretended to read because the person next to me wouldn't stop talking. I looked up from my book and noticed I was the lone African American female patient in this hideout, as I was also on my unit. Maybe it was true that mental illness affected some groups disproportionately more than others. Here inside the hospital, I could see that I was a minority within a minority.

This had to be the only place in the facility where the air conditioner did not reach. It was hot, a tornado we could not see or hear was doing who knows what, and I was only a few days into my mental hospital stint. I never felt my lost freedom more than now. Was my family safe? Had my home been damaged?

Suddenly, the voice on the intercom announced, "All clear!" Just like that, we returned to our unit.

Later, some of us were treated to an outdoor excursion. A few days in the hospital felt like I had never encountered summer breezes, sunbathing, and weeds impersonating flowers. Nature's outside was tickling my insides. An unkempt basketball court was far from the idyllic scenery I'd passed earlier on the way from the emergency room. It didn't matter, because I was happy to be outside.

Our nurse escort found a makeshift stoop to read her book while I settled on a cement step--a few feet away--and did likewise. Some of the men tossed a basketball around, and others just enjoyed a spot of solitude under a shaded tree. Seeing the sky from the outdoors, after days of being locked indoors, was the equivalent of someone touching and tasting snow falling for the first time. It was unmatched and unparalleled, to say the least, and made me empathize with prisoners of any kind, man or animal.

I heard it approaching before I saw it: a familiar sound which was no longer muffled because we were now outside. A passing plane held my attention until all that was left was its faint smoke trail, long after it was out of earshot. Just a year earlier, my daughter and I had the time of our lives flying to San Francisco during an incredibly amazing time. My daughter was being recognized as a scholarship recipient from the Alpha Kappa Alpha Educational Advancement Foundation, Inc. An Alcatraz postcard from this trip hung over my desk at work. I once commented to a coworker how the job felt like an Alcatraz. "At least they can escape," he joked, to which we both grinned.

Fast forward to now and I was watching a plane soar from my spot on the grounds of a psychiatric hospital. *Take me with you. Don't leave me here,* I silently begged as the plane drifted off into the distance. It was interesting how, since my confinement, any part of the outdoors, no matter how unattractive or unreachable, was pleasure in the present. A huge hater of all types of bugs, insects, and spiders, I'd let a bee chase me into a cobweb-- and I wouldn't even scream--if I could bask in the outdoors for just a moment longer. The things you take for granted when your freedom is taken away from you.

Depression had robbed me of so much, including the most basic of things. While in the hospital I was back to sleeping soundly, eating three meals a day, reading leisurely, and enjoying the calming effects of a hot cup of tea every now and again. I didn't want to leave, this place made me feel so special. As one fellow patient said, "Who wants to return to that crappy world?"

There were times when I never wanted to leave my bed, but the staff at the hospital wouldn't leave me alone. Someone was always tugging on me to take medicine, have lab work drawn, talk to clinicians regarding my general health and nutrition, as well as meet with the psychiatrist for my mental health. When they showed up, you would have to make yourself available. No sooner had I retreated to my bed before there'd be someone else to meet, or another place to go. The one time the patient phone was free was same time a doctor was ready to have a conversation. I understood the necessity of a tailored, full, and productive schedule, and not a hospital treatment plan calling for siesta therapy...but still!

I had adapted to the routines of my newfound sanctuary. The therapy sessions, crying to the doctors in sane-face, medicine time, followed by a nightly group trip to the vending machine for my soft and juicy Mike and Ike candy fix--a newly formed, fun habit that may have needed to be addressed and treated. For one habitual smoker in our group, Coke quenched his cigarette cravings until he adjusted to wearing a nicotine patch. With each trip we made in the late evenings through the deserted hospital lobby, we both jockeyed for vending machine position for our sugar vices. We took our comfort wherever we could find it inside the hospital, until we were well enough to be comfortable and functioning on the outside, as discharged patients.

19 *Day Four*

I felt hopeful and rated myself a six on this day, even in the midst of the unknowns and what-ifs. A fire drill interrupted the morning and all I could think was, "Not again!" It was Friday; I was glad to have made it through the first few days in the hospital, when I thought about how I almost didn't cheat death. That was enough to rejoice in the Lord! I still had no plans for my future, other than knowing I had to find a new job.

The end of the week brought in more visitors than usual, and I was granted one of the few conference rooms on the ward to accommodate all of my guests. They included my daughter, one of my former coworkers from a happier job, along with my pastor and his wife. My daughter and I were given Communion when I asked my pastor if he had trouble finding this place I had only recently heard about. He responded that there weren't too many places he didn't know about in our county. That was understandable. Some things shouldn't make it to the list of church announcements, like a congregant taking temporary residence in a mental institution.

As it turned out, one of my ward mates was also a member of my church, and I never knew it until my pastor's visit. It made me wonder how many more people I would encounter who were masking mental illness. Maybe they didn't know exactly what it was they were dealing with. Maybe they thought it would pass and go away on its own. Maybe it was the widely held belief that certain cultures were more resilient to hardships than most, and therefore were not on the radar for mental health assessment and detection.

Whatever my "maybe" was, my certainty was I would not be sharing this story had I not recognized I needed help. I didn't know what I was dealing with, it was not passing and although I knew I was slipping, I continued on as usual, to the best of my natural abilities.

No one is exempt from mental trauma or an emotional meltdown. It hits you like a freight train, rear-ending you and catching you off guard. Everything can change in a split second. But I held on to Jeremiah 29:11 (NKJV) – *"For I know the thoughts that I think toward you, says the Lord, thoughts of peace and not of evil, to give you a future and a hope."* At first there was no light at the end of the tunnel, but now I had no doubt there would be a blessing in this adversity. What was meant for evil would be turned around and used for good (Genesis 50:20, NKJV).

20 *Day Five*

The weekend arrived in what was now known as our "five-star hotel." Due to our similar disorder types, being a patient on our unit came with fewer constraints compared to the other units. Not every unit could dine in the cafeteria along side hospital workers, go outside to play or read, or venture to the vending machines after dark. Walk by any of the other wards and there would be signs of caution. Like any place of business, the hospital was very quiet on the weekends. Instead of being cooped up in the common room, we got to spend our next therapy session outdoors on the café patio.

The social worker that led the session was one we hadn't met before, and the session felt more improvised than scripted; it didn't follow the usual classroom model with the patients reading along from handouts. Spread between two patio tables, my fellow ward mates and I dialogued and shared more about ourselves. I knew mostly everyone's story because everyone freely talked, whether we were in or out of therapy sessions, and I freely eavesdropped while safeguarding my own business. This relaxed formation lowered my defenses enough to share with the group why I had been admitted.

It was not genetics or an addiction disorder, like it was for some, but it was a curve ball thrown my way that made direct impact with my very existence, unraveling every chord and pulse that kept me alive. My life, leading up to my hospitalization, was like a pinball machine. The pinball game ended when the ricocheting steel ball destroyed all of the targets. No more dings, blasts, or lights. "Game over!" flashed across the backboard. The game's playfield had been deserted, becoming a mute ghost of what it used to be at the peak of its playing action. I was not who I used to be. The vibrant life I once lived had deserted me and left me alone with depression. I came from an acrimonious work environment that was run by an out of control, ball of steel - a manager who targeted my life for destruction, until my life would cease. *"Life over!"*

I remembered the screening questions regarding my social habits and past history. My answers indicated all was stable, normal, and copacetic. Childhood and family dynamics? Good. Substance abuse, alcohol, and addictive behaviors? None. Education and work background? Superb. Psychiatric history? Nonexistent. At the conclusion of the psychosocial assessment, the clinical social worker said I was the perfect patient.

Since becoming a mental health patient I've learned that, according to some experts, African Americans tend to be depressed because social class, racial oppression, poverty, and economics have roles in our mental health. I was middle class and educated, breaking the African American mental patient mold right from the jump. Considering I was also a Christian and an active member of a church body, which by most accounts should have made me depression proof, and I further shattered that mold into a million pieces.

There was one lifestyle that made me predisposed for depression, according to some studies: I was a single parent. My worst day as a single parent was better than my best day in an abusive marriage, so I imagine I've completely thrown off the research data and boosted the margin of error. This mild-mannered mother of two, with no prior mental health history, lived an occasionally challenging yet happy life overall until I was aided and abetted into a state of worthlessness and suicidal thoughts by a bully. My supervisor drove me insane, and that's why I had been admitted.

My confession to the group came without coercion or being asked, bringing relief for what up until then had only been revealed to staff, family, and close friends. All was quiet as they listened. My tears had taken a break but when all was said and done, my fellow patients rallied to my defense, having known me for less than a week. This time, I wasn't offended by the cursing and the things they called management; on the contrary, they assured me it wasn't my fault that I landed in the hospital. In solidarity, they put aside their own issues and had my back.

When the session leader asked what would I have done differently leading up to my crisis, I replied that I would have sought treatment sooner, now that I had a better understanding of depression. I was the head of my household with children depending on me, and always had to maintain a strong front and suppress any pain to buffer and protect my family. I didn't think I was permitted to be downcast.

Later that evening, I finished reading *The Island of Dr. Moreau*. The ward's makeshift library offerings were slim to none but based on the tattered, dingy condition of my choice, this book must have been the original 1896 publication. I was twelve years old when I first saw the movie in theaters, starring Burt Lancaster. I'm not sure why my aunt let me pick this movie for our movie date or why I had chosen it, for that matter. But I never forgot the film, or the time spent with my favorite aunt. Aunt Louise was legally blind but that never hindered her from a life of loving and giving. I adored her and it could have been coming across that book in the hospital reminded me of a more beautiful and innocent time.

What was not beautiful were some of the book's themes – tyranny, exploitation, and immorality; abuse, pain and suffering; conflict, despair, and death; misguided faith and playing God. It nearly read like my current situation. The island hybrids escaped from captivity and returned to normalcy when the villain was exterminated. If only I could have eliminated my abuser to get my normal back.

The average length of stay for a patient on my unit was four to six days. My time in the hospital, sadly, was winding down. The hospital's role was to alleviate my suicidal crisis and stabilize me enough, so that I could transition to outpatient treatment for a full recovery and long-term wellness. These mental health care

Samaritans rescued my mind, but it would take a lot of time before my mind could be nursed back to its former state of bliss. I prayed for God to keep me in His perfect peace, and sustain my tranquility these remaining nights in the hospital.

21 *The Mind Savers*

Depression, and taking up residence inside a psychiatric hospital, were foreign to me. I owed my life to mental health care professionals who devoted themselves to taking care of people like me, people lost in translation, whose lives mattered and were worthy to be lived.

I heard a saying in the Baptist church that went something like this: either you were called to preach...or you were crazy. I felt that mental health care workers had answered a calling. You couldn't work in this field if you didn't truly care about making people well. It's not an occupation to enter just to pay the bills. It required your dedication and your heart.

The social worker leading the majority of our sessions--a minister by trade--kept us enlightened by sharing aspects from her personal life with such transparency, we felt like she was our best friend and didn't want her to leave us at the end of each day. "You matter because you were born," was her mantra. She was dedicated to us, and we adored her.

Then there were the nursing students on rotation from the local community college, who would sit in on our group sessions and observe. I sometimes wondered if mental health was off the career table after they'd listened to our tales from the dark side for an hour. I spoke to one of the students after a session and asked if depression was prevalent in his country. I couldn't recall which

African country he called home, but he explained that depression was fairly nonexistent where he was from, as people were generally content with their lives. He then asked how I came to be in the hospital. His question didn't bother me, and I answered. Because he was only observing and not a member of my treatment team, it may have been an inappropriate question. Nevertheless, I understood how I'd be a curiosity to some if you weren't used to seeing African American women as patients in psychiatric hospitals. Anyone could be susceptible to mental illness, but not everyone had the health insurance--like I did--to be treated in a good mental facility.

My mental health journey wouldn't be complete without my betrothal to a psychiatrist. Contrary to what I'd seen on television, I wouldn't be reclining on a sofa, unloading all my problems to a pen and pad-holding man in a white shirt and tie. The ward, when busy, looked and felt like a major downtown metropolitan area. Private meetings with the psychiatrist took place wherever there was space, even if it was in the utility closet. Meetings could happen at any time: not long after I awoke, or right when I was ready to go to bed for the night.

My assigned psychiatrist happened to be the medical director of the behavioral health center. All eyes were on me as I recited again, for two lab coat-wearing interns and a Phil Jackson look-alike of average height, why I was there. More tears, more anguish reliving what was still fresh trauma. Then silence. *What we have here is failure to communicate, Cool Hand Doc.* Not one note was taken by the doctor and the best poker face I had ever seen, divulged nothing. The doctor kept a Diet Coke next to him and caressed his cell phone most of the time; yes, he talked to me while looking at his phone. I answered some questions and then the meeting quickly ended. It was draining, rehashing the same ugly events.

Tears ran often to fill the long pauses in between the doctor's few comments. "You're still rocking," was one of them. It was a habit I hadn't noticed each time we'd talk. He actually brought it to my attention one meeting, leading me to believe he was observing much more than I thought. If my mind wasn't so weak, I would have used my Wonder Twin superhero powers to morph into a dove and fly away to a happy place. I had no one to "fist bump" to activate my transforming powers, therefore the best my altered state of mind could do--as I sat with my psychiatrist-- was to take the form of a rocking chair. The imagination could be a playful thing, but it wasn't a superhero fantasy that made me rock in place. Rocking was a natural reaction to being traumatized, and there was nothing playful about that.

The interns also had conditioned poker faces. Three sets of eyes all on me, looking through me, analyzing me. Sometimes we were crammed so tight in our meeting spot our knees touched from our seated positions. Even after I said (while still rocking) I wanted to shoot my boss dead if only I had a gun, I could have just as well said it was sunny today. The three didn't flinch, blink, or respond. They were internally, surveying with my mind--when it seemed to me they were calmly waiting to see if I would fold my poker hand, call the bet, or raise. *Twirl a pencil, shift in your seat, clear your throat--say something, damn it!* It was all in a day's work for psychiatrists.

The weekends were slightly different. The ward was quieter without the distractions of the weekday hustle and bustle. The doctor on weekend duty was not one of our regular psychiatrists. Meh was my impression of her. The fact she was female didn't sway me to think I'd have a softer meeting.

I had been summoned by the previous patient who saw the stand-in psychiatrist, and was told that she wanted to see me. *Tag, you're it.* Usually an intern came for me, if my psychiatrist did not. Holed up in the large conference room behind a rolling cart filled with our unit's patient records (mine was in her hands), the weekend psychiatrist was closer to my age and without an intern entourage. She was also without her cell phone in plain view.

It was easy to notice the doctor's slow and steady breathing, as she took her time flipping through the pages of my chart. I looked around the conference room, fidgeting in my seat, until she was ready to talk to me.

I answered her questions, offering very little commentary except wondering about my job safety after my discharge. She told me I could hire a labor attorney. Then our session was over. I found the next patient and told him the psychiatrist was ready to see him. *Tag, you're it.*

Stabilizing antidepressants were prescribed and adjusted to match my mood disorder as the crisis that peaked days earlier started to retreat. Wonder Twin powers, deactivate! Form of: the life I had before the meltdown.

I gained a tremendous amount of respect for mental health care professionals. To me they were saints, providing care to those easily ostracized in society. I considered them the Mother Teresas and Florence Nightingales of the health profession. War veterans, nurses, and teachers have always been my heroes. Now I added mental health professionals to the list.

22 *Day Six*

That day's session involved an exercise naming the one thing we liked about ourselves and did not want to change. Patients in the group took turns giving their responses and when I answered how I liked and would not change my heart, others didn't hesitate to chime in and concur. Finally, a real smile on the outside! It was a defining moment to have my peers confer such an accolade, having known me for less than a week. I had been so used to being the bull's eye for management's dysfunctional dart-throwing pleasure, and in the thick of all kinds of depravity for so long, that it warmed my soul when my hospital family saw a decent person, good heart, and beautiful human spirit almost right away. I was grateful that I had earned their admiration and respect.

Months of working under a bully had critically wounded my self-esteem, but this human vessel had not become a byproduct of management's wickedness. I was God's property and it showed. He still gleamed from the inside out. While my mind may have been momentarily captured, I thanked God for guarding my heart.

Being cared for in a faith-based hospital allowed me to attend worship service on Sunday. This type of facility--which cared for the physical, emotional, and spiritual needs of every patient--was crucial to my healing. At the time of my admission, however, I didn't care what type of facility was going to treat me. I was too depressed to think about my religious foundation while I was preparing to take my life. It was fortunate that this particular hospital was close to my home, especially when there were two nationally ranked mental institutions (that were not faith-based) only an hour's drive away. The mere fact I was still alive had me wanting to praise God. I had already come to depend on the morning devotionals shared over the intercom system throughout the week and was now ready for church which, like everything else, required a staff escort.

The sermon came from the parable of the Great Banquet in Luke 14:15-24. In the parable, well-to-do guests were invited to feast at the table but declined. The invites then went out to the downtrodden, where these guests filled the house and feasted. God's kingdom was open to anyone willing to come.

While getting ready for management's death squad one morning, I took a detour to the hospital instead and, in a week, was rewarded with lifelong lessons and a spot at the table. God saved my life when I didn't think my life was worth living. This was my testimony to the other patients attending service.

23 *Day Seven*

My morning self-ratings had been hovering between six and seven. Who gives a ten rating in a mental institution? Had I received word the agency finally believed me, dismissed my manager, worked to undo all his wrongs in my personnel file, and pushed full steam ahead to assure this would never happen to anyone else again, I would have been a 100.

New arrivals replaced patients who had been discharged over the last few days, and I had a room to myself following my roommate's release. Throughout our time together on the ward, Princess and I came to an understanding without speaking a word, and that's how I liked it. She stayed to herself, and I stayed to myself. I was now roommate-less and loving it, but soon a new patient arrived on a stretcher. She had flawless dreads and skin so perfect; I had only seen similar skin on newborns and doctored photos. Most of us arrived ambulatory, or by wheelchair. This was a first I'd seen a patient delivered to the ward on a stretcher.

We all thought I had a new roommate, but then we soon discovered the latest addition to our island of misfit minds was actually male and looked young enough to be in high school. I wondered why he'd been admitted, and speculated on the cause. Had he been bullied as well? It was bad enough having to deal with one monster but when you had multiple bullies, one continuing where the previous bully left off, I could only imagine you would be a repeat inpatient, if not a suicide success story.

With my discharge approaching, I wouldn't get to spend a lot of time with the young man whom we initially thought was a female. But from what I knew of him, he was all right with me. Soft-spoken and always one to hold the door open for a lady, Gentle Ben quickly earned my admiration over some of the goons I had lived with for the past week. We were a family but when it came time to eat, the men climbed to the front of the chow line and left the women at the end of the line. Not Gentle Ben. He had the traits of a perfect gentleman, a refreshing sight to see when people these days were so cruel.

I was happy when he joined me for a game of Uno. Reverse, skip, and draw were now replaced with action symbols with meanings Gentle Ben had to explain to me, since the last time I played Uno was probably before he was born. Later, I asked him to join us for a game of Spades but he confessed he hadn't quite gotten the hang of it from watching us play. When I reflect back on my time spent in the hospital, he would be the one patient I would always wonder about.

The one patient I planned not to think about again would be Ms. Thornbird, my replacement roommate. She, too, came in on a stretcher but after a few minutes, walked into the common room where we all were.

"Who's Lisa?" she asked.

"I'm Lisa," I replied in a defensive tone that said, "*Is there a problem?*"

"Oh, you're my roommate!"

I hope Ms. Thornbird wasn't expecting me to jump up and down and shout "hooray!" Suddenly, I missed Princess. We may not have had much in common, but we were both respectfully quiet, compared to Ms. Thornbird. I must have made a face unwittingly because I looked over to see one of the guys across the room, smirking at me. I was never good at hiding my facial expressions.

She was the only patient to come in chirping right away. Others were withdrawn and quiet until they had acclimated, like I had been. It could've been because she was a repeat admission. Ms. Thornbird noisily strolled around the common room--picking up objects and observing them--like she was on a guided tour. Occasionally, she would stop moving to reminisce; it appeared she liked being back in the hospital. She noticed nothing had changed since her last stay, as if she was laying claim to previously marked territory. Ordinarily I'm an even keel, mellow fellow, speaker of few words, mind-my-own-business, impose not kinda gal, and my inpatient stay hadn't changed that. The new roommate was anything but, and was an annoyance very early.

She talked a lot and was too intrusive, asking me about my medications, wandering onto my nightstand to touch my artwork, invading the rest of my personal space, and sharing with me what should have been told to her doctor. Had we bunked together on day one, I would've been placed in solitary confinement for a misdemeanor. Intermingling and camaraderie had their places, but not at that point and time. After all, I was a patient too and frankly, I didn't like her or care about her issues. My hiding places were limited so I tuned her out by hiding my face in a book, escaping to a different area, or dosing out on insomnia meds just so I could fall asleep on her while she chatted on into the night.

Soon I'd be leaving, but soon couldn't arrive fast enough. What remained was the family meeting, which reminded me of a parole board hearing to determine if I would be fit to reenter society as a positive contributor, rather than as a mental delinquent. Inside these walls, I felt safe. I was unsure about the outside.

24 *Coming to the End of One Journey*

Being a psychiatric inpatient was not all group sessions and psychiatrist meetings. While not mandatory, recreational therapy created a diversion to residual negative thoughts. There were some activities I would never have tried outside of the hospital. They weren't something to get excited about because they were on the schedule, but incorporating them into a day broke the monotony and filled empty minutes when a book or television programming wouldn't do.

Yoga would be one of those activities I'd only do under a doctor's orders. Because it was offered, I tried it and would be the only pupil this day. While I appreciated the ambience of Tibetan nature sounds and the tranquility of flute lullabies, what I didn't appreciate was the wafer-thin mat/tile floor combination sabotaging my knees and spine. When the class was over, there was no part of my body that didn't ache. Yoga failed to deliver the peace it promised. When the class rotated back around, I declined. In my stead were two young male patients who seemed to enjoy themselves. They did much better holding yoga stances than I did; they looked like they were interlocked in a game of Twister. A game spinner and a large plastic mat with colored circles were all that were needed to make me chuckle at these men.

There was also a music class. Unlike yoga, the music session was standing room only. For forty-five minutes I learned the difference between two types of guitars; I just don't remember what those differences were. As the other patients took turns strumming away at what was not music to my ears, my mood to pluck guitar strings took a rain check. What I wanted the instructor to do was play the opening guitar solo to Prince's "When Doves Cry." Other patients barked out commands as well. We must have made him feel like the cheap entertainment for a bachelor party. He declined to entertain us; he was there to teach us music and take our minds off our problems for a spell.

Whether yoga or music, paid or volunteer, it made you wonder who would sign on to interact with adults who had mental health challenges. The instructor shared how he used to visit children with cancer but became distraught when he would return, only to find out that a child had passed away. That told me he wasn't just doing a job, he was working from the soul. I commended him, and others like him, for offering to help us heal.

Next to journaling, art allowed me to purge and was my favorite of all the therapies. I couldn't draw a lick, but something about taking markers and bringing a black-and-white outline to life felt good.

She was only a shell when I deliberately chose her over the other outlines. Truth was she noticed me first and didn't need my purple and gold strokes to define her being. It was obvious she already had worth, purpose, and beauty. The outline suggested she came from royalty; perhaps she was an Egyptian princess. An internet search later revealed she was a queen: she was Nefertiti, and she was me. I named my coloring "ROYALTY" and added the inscription, "*I am royalty. I am a daughter, sister, mother, and friend.*" I studied my colored interpretive expression that a three year-old Picasso would've outdrawn, and held it at eye level to make sure I had left no area uncolored. On a separate piece of poster paper I etched these words –

I want to live.

I want my joy back.

You did not have the right to steal my joy.

I am somebody, and I am loved.

One of the final exercises as an inpatient was to describe what changes we had made since coming to the hospital. My answer was my perspective on mental health and depression. Depression was nothing to take lightly, and could be linked to suicidal or homicidal ideation. It abducted my thoughts where I no longer registered what was sane and sensible. While real to me, my world seemed deranged to anyone else. Empathy was useless unless you had lost yourself in depression, and didn't care if you were ever found.

I felt that sadness and depression were distant relatives. Sadness had a faster recovery. If it were an infection, an antibiotic could kill it and have you back to normal. It was like wearing a coat in the winter but removing the coat in the summer because the season had changed. Sadness was the red or green light of a traffic signal, the on/off switch of a device. It could stop or go readily, or be turned off as quickly as it was turned on.

Depression, on the other hand, was the yellow light. It didn't know stopping for red was momentary, and eventually life could proceed again on green. The coat that came off in the summer remained on through all four seasons because you were unaware the weather had changed. The infection that was treatable before, had now proliferated into a virus that defied conventional medicines, hiding in your DNA and prone to reemerge with certain triggers. Depression, I'd say, was sadness on steroids and took on a life of its own. It made me feel like I was under house arrest, only there was no house.

25 *Depression, Anyone?*

Before I was admitted to the hospital for depression, I remembered wishing for an ailment. Desperate times called for desperate measures, and a depressed mind had desperate thoughts. I wanted anything that could get me out of going to work, something that was easy to diagnose and highly treatable. I knew better than to wish for cancer but I thought about it, a one-time depressing thought. Little did I know I would fall to mental illness several months later and, by doing so be protected by health care professionals whose duty it was to keep me well by upholding standards of medical ethics. No respectable medical service provider would compromise my health by returning me to work in a place that claimed my mental wellness. That would be like prescribing cigarettes to an emphysema patient.

Imagine how stunned I was when my psychiatrist asked what was I going to do about the job. His question had me fuming, trembling, and hyperventilating all in one motion. "I can't go back there! If I do, someone's not going to live!" Why would he ask such a question, knowing what that job did to me? I now believe it was just an assessment question to gauge my rationality. That's when the psychiatrist mentioned disability. I'd worked since I was a teenager - 10,950 days accident-free. Now I was impaired for the first time in my working career.

It was not the escape route I envisioned, but it was the one God provided. I would be free from the job, but at the cost of acquiring a mental disability. I was conflicted in my faith because my spirituality didn't suppress the depression. I felt that I was a disappointing example of a worshiping Christian, and my faith grade was a large capital F circled in red. Nothing I prayed, meditated on, studied in bible classes, or listened to musically for a gospel uplift helped me during those dismal workdays. My mind had been held hostage and was brainwashed with unfamiliar thoughts invading my place of innermost peace and safety, thoughts I couldn't discern. They visited me with the frequency of uterine contractions just prior to a newborn's first breath. Now I understood why my spirit couldn't be consoled: I was dangerously depressed and didn't realize it, believing all along I was just unhappy.

A new job I thought held promise for elevating me to the top of my profession, delivered me to the front door of a psychiatric hospital, instead. The moment I crossed the threshold, I became a mental patient. Having no history of mental illness, I suffered from the effects of depression and anxiety but unintentionally masked it. That's what makes depression such an insidious bastard, a bully in and of itself. It gives the appearance nothing is out of the ordinary until your loved ones are left puzzled, trying to figure out how in the blink of an eye you killed yourself.

I didn't wake up with a plan to take my life that day. It was an impulse as soon as my daughter left for work and I was alone. Eradicating depression meant calling on suicide for help. Would I have taken a fatal dose, or would I have toyed with a few pills, thinking I would have been found in time to be saved? I wondered how many people thought the latter, miscalculated the number of pills, and did not make it. The answer will never be known.

Since I didn't know anything about depression, I was oblivious to the changes I'd been going through. Withdrawing socially; losing weight; declining interest in hobbies and activities; ignoring the upkeep of my home and myself; sleeping a lot or not sleeping at all; and sulking daily were the telltale signs and symptoms I had arrived at depression's front door. I became its favorite house guest and roommate before ultimately tying the knot and giving birth to twins: homicidal and suicidal thoughts.

Once freed and placed into protective custody of the hospital where my mind and body would be reinvigorated, I discovered I was the textbook example of depression. Depression had infiltrated and seized the vines of my cerebral cortex, something I expected dementia to do when I aged another thirty years. I was so close to death; I fell over the ledge of suicide's cliff but miraculously, the mercy workers of behavioral healthcare broke my fall.

About this time, were news headlines nationwide reporting on stories with a common denominator: depression led suicide among African Americans. They were celebrities, successful entrepreneurs, and just everyday people. And yes, some were even pastors. Not only were some of the sheep (such as myself) battling mental illness, but also the shepherds--the pastors who were anointed to lead God's flock. Had anyone told me I'd be treated for mental illness a few years shy of fifty, and midway through my government career, I would have never believed them.

I also wouldn't have believed I'd be inside a psychiatric hospital. In a time when there was an increased awareness for being respectful, inclusive, and nondiscriminatory, I spent time in a psychiatric hospital called by another name. You may find that either "psychiatric" is omitted from the institution's name, or it has been most likely replaced with "behavioral." Thank God these institutions existed, no matter what they were called, for the purpose of treating broken minds.

God's grace and favor got me through many tests and trials before. Anger, sure. Bitterness, absolutely. These were expected feelings from life beating you up from time to time. Then came something that broke my resilience and placed me in a club whose dues were paid with mindless bias and lifetime stigma--the depression club. It wouldn't matter if my disorder was situational or genetic; a single occurrence, or reoccurring. I acquired all of the prejudices that went along with it, no matter how it originated. As a newly diagnosed client of mental illness, I was forever branded. Membership would be for a lifetime.

"Hello, my name is Lisa and I'm a mental health patient." This was my truth, and don't think for a minute it couldn't be yours too. I'm not ashamed of acquiring a psychiatric disability, because I'm too grateful to God for simply being alive.

26 *Day Eight*

Another day, a closer step to being dressed in my right mind. My health took quite a blow when depression changed my life. The wounds were still fresh, but at least I felt better a week later, while still in treatment. It must have been evident because the nurse giving me my nightly medicine told me I looked so much better, as did my psychiatrist.

When I first came through the doors of the mental hospital, I looked like I'd been through hell - the kind of hell I remembered from a scene in the movie *What's Love Got to Do with It*. Tina Turner's character, played by Angela Bassett, fled to a hotel after a bloody and fierce fight with Ike Turner's character, played by Laurence Fishburne. Explaining her dilemma to the manager on duty, she removed her jewelry as payment for a stay but the manager refused it. She was assured that wasn't necessary and she'd be taken care of. The manager could clearly tell from the swollen bruises and fresh scars that she had been in a battle. The mental war waged inside me felt like this defining movie scene; I wore the scars that were quite noticeable, from an internal battle no one could see.

I was glad that others noticed my progress. The medication and therapy were working. The crisis was over! Each patient arrived on the unit emotionally spent and scarred. It looked as if we had been dragged from beneath the earth when we were deposited into a sanctuary for missing and exploited minds. Some were first-timers and others repeaters, but we all wanted to be well and were each other's keepers.

I once went to the gym not because I had a desire to work out, but because a patient who really wanted to get off the ward and shoot some hoops asked me. The supervised outing required at least one more patient, and no one else wanted to go. I brought along a book to read and he got in his workout. The favor was returned when the US Open Championship took a break for a day while I got to watch what I wanted for once, the Miami Heat – San Antonio Spurs basketball game. Wrapping up a game of cards, I moved from the table and took over the TV chair, that one off-angled chair that belonged with the table but was tilted to view the TV. There I sat, tuning out all the other activity and noise in the common room. It was just me and Spurs legend Tim Duncan, professionally known also as "The Big Fundamental." No one else cared for San Antonio; they were pro-Miami, but at least I got to enjoy the game and some me time without being bothered by anyone else. These were the types of things we did for one another.

If one was down, we would take turns consoling and cheering him or her because we were caring humans regardless of our ailments, almost getting to the point of anger someone would think so low of himself or herself when we saw otherwise. I remembered the first time I laughed while inside the psychiatric hospital, although it never showed on the outside because depression had my joy on lockdown. It was when I once overheard a patient say, "Man, my great grandfather looked like freakin' Colonel Sanders. Seriously, with the bow tie and everything!" That image evolved in my head and made me erupt in laughter, no one else heard.

Tiny, the one patient making a scene at the nurses' station when I first arrived turned out to be harmless. She was a pest to most of the other patients and was yelled at or shooed away more than a bad first date seeking a second date. We all had disorders we were trying to combat and most couldn't be bothered with the extra attention she wanted, too. Unlike others, I had to look beyond Tiny's quirks and engage her like she was a child. Apparently it must have worked, because she seemed to take to me.

We were where we needed to be for healing but when it was time to be discharged, we couldn't wait to post bail and get out of our "jail." Every discharge was a happy one; you took your last walk around the unit, going room to room dispensing goodbyes, good lucks, huge smiles, and long hugs. We had been revived and the lives we almost took had been recharged to break bad habits, dump unhealthy relationships, and just live, man...just live. I prayed a full and continued recovery for each patient leaving, wanting each to have the best life had to offer so no one would ever come back.

They brought wisdom, insight, and value to the mix, even those who were initially scary. There was the California Surfer, the Philosopher, Mr. Charisma, the Golfer, Dilbert, Raven, Princess, Ms. Thornbird, Tiny, Gentle Ben, and Scarface – the code names I had secretly given to a few of the patients. What I appreciated was Mr. Charisma commenting in one of our last group sessions how Dilbert and I were smiling for the first time. I wasn't the only one with a good heart in our group. At the beginning of the week, I had been ready to die and got locked away with strangers. What was there to smile about? By the end of that week, though, I was sure I wanted to live; that was worth several smiles!

There would be no new BFFs, Facebook connections, or Instagram follows. What happened on the ward, stayed on the ward. The patients I'd met were mostly forgotten as I prepared for life on the outside.

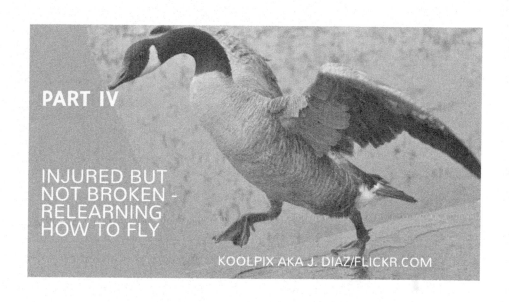

PART IV

**INJURED BUT
NOT BROKEN -
RELEARNING
HOW TO FLY**

27 *The Right HELP!*

My medical crisis was a rallying cry for the saints and prayer warriors in my life. An emergency alert was issued for Healing through Encouragement, Love, and Prayer (HELP). My happiness had been abducted, hope held ransom, and will to live depleted. HELP would come from all over as word spread I had contemplated suicide because of a job, a bully, a hater.

After months of being the object of contempt and ill will, it was nice to finally be nurtured with every prayer call received, tender card written, house call made, and fellowship outing taken. There was no shortage of never-ending good deeds by kind people who did what they were called to do when someone was weak and wounded. They donned their spiritual hero capes of compassion and selflessness to be of service; some even offered to donate their vacation days so I'd have some income for what was going to be a very long road to recovery. I would have done the same.

"Grateful" would be an understatement, yet it was still not easy to receive and even harder to ask for help. My daughters and I had been the recipients of many random acts of kindness following my divorce. But for the goodness then of family, friends, church members, coworkers, supervisors, strangers, and nonprofits, we never went hungry and always had a place to live.

Life's vulnerable events helped plant the seed over twenty years ago to always think of others who were having as tough a time. I raised my family on this foundation. I humbly say this was a testament to how we lived. And it was returned with interest when caring people were willing to go the extra mile to accompany me on my healing odyssey. Had I been a cantankerous or unsavory type of person, I may not have gotten the same outpouring of HELP. How are you living, and how do people see you? If suddenly you were down on your luck, would HELP quickly come your way? I believe how I lived was a direct reflection of the extraordinary and beautiful HELP I received. I would have perished otherwise.

28 *The New Untouchables*

A few bad supervisors wanted to incapacitate employees, rendering them cripple, insane, and unable to function. If this dysfunctional environment appealed to you, then apply within at my agency. It would be rare, if not impossible, to find any agency's mission and vision marketing such a philosophy; but this is what management was allowed to do to me. If my agency couldn't have cared less about me and what I went through under their manager, then they had to care about the bottom line: as in, paying wages for no productivity because of my extended leave of absence.

Nothing felt worse than having my own agency turn its back on me. My complaints fell on disobliging ears, which then made me a prime target for further abuse until my mental health gave way. To have them tell it, the stars were misaligned in the galaxies, which created a disturbance that propelled a loony meteorite down to earth which landed smack dead in the middle of my forehead, controlling my mind. Seriously? Just let me dust off my Atari 5200 system, lock and load some Asteroids into the game console, and zap the little buggers to keep them from sucking me into the fifth dimensional mental black hole again!

Workers beware! If only "worker's remorse" existed and allowed us to make a hasty exit from a job we regretted accepting. We could then return to the safe retreat of a former job with no questions asked. Had I known beforehand what I was getting into, I would have never left a job where I was content. If consumers can make an educated spending decision after researching the profile, ratings, and service history of any business, then why isn't there a Better Bosses Bureau available for rating managers before a job candidate accepts a position? Is the US Department of Labor ready to publically disclose the number of complaints a manager has on record, and if any of those complaints resulted in high turnover, employee injury, or legal action? Analytics won't lie, and transparency could save lives.

If someone could kill with just a look, I would have died a thousand times over. My manager's hate for me was that palpable, as if I was an offensive odor he couldn't stand to be around. Working for him felt like I was a ward of the state to a wicked foster parent who only saw me as a monthly check, and would readily kill me just to keep collecting money under false pretenses. In work terms, I was no more to my manager than a budget line item, a number to boost his operating expenses, greed, power, and facade with no investment in my professional development and success. Instead, I was used for everything he could squeeze out of me for his own credit and ego. The fact that I lasted as long as I did under such a regime and lived to talk about it was astonishing. I deserved a medal!

Management had no right, as an agency representative in his official duties, to inflict injury upon his employee. If this was allowed, despite strong assertions that were never investigated and now medical evidence attesting to major depressive disorder (MDD) with post-traumatic stress disorder (PTSD), then this kind of supervisor was not competent to lead--particularly at an agency voted as one of the top places to work. My boss had the authority to get away with behaving badly and the agency called it appropriate supervising. They saw no evil, heard no evil, and spoke no evil when it came to their golden boy, a bad seed that I almost de-germinated.

Prior complaints trailed my supervisor like an oil slick in the ocean. By the time I put Employee Relations on notice about him, alarms, sirens, and whistles should have gone off. Had the agency pooled together all of these complaints and assessed them over time, they could have intercepted my manager before things got out of hand. Common sense should have trumped by-the-book sense, but it didn't because you had an agency policing itself. Had this been a matter between two peers instead of between a supervisor and supervisee, it may have been handled in a manner far more conducive to unbiased arbitration, leading to coherent solutions for working respectfully and amicably between the ranks.

Advising a worker to find another job doesn't address a detestable manager. His unlikableness cannot be written off as a character flaw to ignore, work around, and accept if he's making workers sick, nearly to the point of death. He will use that same murderous leadership on each successor. Management privilege overruled subordinate fairness and justice, in my case. This was the new Good Ol' Boys network, where higher ranks were protected while lower ranks were ignored. Had my injury been the result of a physical assault, this story would have had a different ending; for I can only believe the job would have stepped in to promptly handle the situation, even if it meant bringing in law enforcement. Why should an emotional assault be any different, especially since it required treatment in a hospital?

What was gained from losing an employee to hostile leadership? An acquired medical disability, leading to claims filed, lawsuits considered, negative publicity garnered, and rising turnover, not to mention low morale for those who were witnesses and remained under such leadership. My boss knew he assigned more work than one person could manage; I could not keep up. For that type of work environment, the world's greatest superheroes would not have been up to par. I saved copies of the emails for myself as proof, but my agency warned me that the emails belonged to them, establishing the notion that my well-being was secondary to digital property.

There's something to be said about departing an agency on a stretcher after decades of unblemished service. My supervisor had a pass to assassinate my character and destroy my will through lies and intimidation, with no oversight or accountability. This meant that the policies and practices of this agency were diseased and forced workers into states of debilitating crises, some who sadly could succumb to death. How many more workers will be treated for professional depression due to jobs not known for being depression-prone occupations, before Houston realizes we've got a problem here? Welcome to the cure, a survivor of workplace bullying who would bring what had been kept on the down low out into the open.

My supervisor was a master of premeditated treachery. His method of operation was ingenious and deliberately sinister. He either tormented you until you resigned, or set you up for insubordination or incompetence for a justifiable termination. I would not be his first. It was Basic Retaliation 101, a course the agency failed to take. His ways for driving me crazy had no bounds.

He had reiterated for months how inept I was, and he constantly voiced his dissatisfaction with my work performance. In spite of his low opinion of me, this did not stop him from overloading me with new assignments that suddenly became urgent and due immediately.

Unhappy that I didn't report to work during a hurricane, my manager changed my status from non-essential to essential. Now I was required to report to work during weather related closings and federal government shutdowns to perform tasks that were deemed "critical" to the group's operations. My job was not related to public health, safety, welfare, or key operations. He wanted me to come in just to do a routine's day of work that was urgent only to him. Surely, I wasn't made essential because of my supervisor's high regard and respect for my skills.

If you took a sick day off, my boss made you bring in a doctor's note before you could return to work. When it came time for vacations, he would only allow you to take five consecutive days off at a time. I do not know why he denied vacation requests that exceeded five days, like the one time I asked for six days and was turned down. You would have thought he'd be happy to let an "underperforming" employee take all the time she wanted if she was a liability to the group.

Toward the end of my time under my manager's reign, I was given an "important" project that required skills I had not learned. "If you were qualified, you'd know what to do," my manager would tell me when I asked for help. Since when does being unqualified mean sentencing an employee to a psychiatric death? Who gives the most important assignments to the "weakest" worker? The answer is a bully who was turning assignments into punishment.

I lived through it and am telling what I know. My manager wanted to do away with an employee whose only crime was exposing his wrongdoing. It became convenient for him to say I wasn't qualified. The agency could not see this but my medical team did, even though they were not present on my job. They merely treated the after effects of what management had done.

Had the outcome been different and my illness became severe enough that I ended up murdering people on the job, society would have considered me disturbed while my family would be lobbying for a Lisa's Law to give workers more protection against workplace bullying. A costly investigation would have pointed to a dishonest manager. Case closed, story grows old, and life goes on.

My manager showed no concern for me at all, after he found out I'd been in the hospital. One of the last communications I had from him caught me by surprise. It was the first time he'd contacted me since I'd fallen ill. He emailed me--as I lay on my recovery bed--with details of the work I'd left incomplete, comments on how unsatisfactory my performance had been, and what tasks to expect upon my return to work. He also reminded me that the deadlines he imposed before my hospitalization, were still in effect.

I knew exactly why the man who was responsible for my illness, had contacted me that day: he was angry about the workers' compensation claim I'd filed the day before. As my supervisor, he was the first to review my claim; it required his signature. I detailed the abuse and exposed his treachery. He didn't appreciate that because the very next day, he sent the email. There was no reason for my boss to send me details of any work assignments while I was on an official leave of absence; he already knew I'd be off from work for most of the year.

I wasn't surprised that he would send such an email. It was the same bullying tactics I'd endured all along. Whenever I complained, he dumped more work on me. Because I wasn't physically on the job to harass, he did the next thing he could--he planted the workload in my mind to achieve the same disturbing effects. It didn't work. There was no way in hell I'd ever return to work for him! What I couldn't believe was how stupid he was to send the email. In a moment of retaliation, he proved I had been telling the truth about him. What kind of supervisor would injure his worker and then tell her she still had work to do? The kind who was cynical, cold, and calculating.

If you were looking for integrity it would not be found in this manager. In fact anything he says should be treated with caution, as with any report he's submitted or paper he's published. We've got a criminal here, one who would even lie on my workers' compensation claim when he stated that he was unaware that the job was making me sick. I told him so! He refused to adjust my workload, or modify my assignments. How unscrupulous can you be when you'd willfully make an untrue statement on a federal form? Can we have a prosecution please, along with an agency shakedown?

A manager representing a government agency tried to kill me. It's as plain and simple as that. In our tense, brief working relationship, we despised one another. I hated him because he represented all things evil. He hated me because I did not. While my feelings were suppressed for fear of a fine, suspension, or termination, his feelings would escalate to overt bullying with no regard for human life. I now carry the mental scars from my supervisor's wrath and, as a result, have a psychiatric rap sheet long enough to make anyone think I've been treated for mental illness since I was born. Have a roundtable discussion with psychiatrists who are treating abused workers and let the data on bullying facts speak for itself. Better yet, open up a poll of one question: "Have you ever been bullied by a supervisor?" See how many hits you'll get in the first day.

I had the right to come to work without fear. The agency had an obligation to protect me. Bullying on the job will pay for itself either in death or dollars from lives lost and pecuniary damages. Only then would managers no longer enjoy impunity.

For we do not wrestle against flesh and blood, but against principalities, against powers, against the rulers of the darkness of this age, against spiritual hosts of wickedness in the heavenly places. Therefore take up the whole armor of God, that you may be able to withstand in the evil day, and having done all, to stand.

Ephesians 6:12-13 (NKJV)

29 *Am I Free?*

Unseen, but not undetectable, described the feeling of stepping inside my home the first time after I'd been discharged from the mental facility. I was met with genuine, authentic peace and calm, as if I had walked into another dimension and the prior week in the hospital never happened. I stood still to bask in what was surely the beauty of God's presence, my body relaxing from the embrace of my omnipotent Host. The house had not changed; it looked just as it did before I was admitted. It showed no signs of the life-and-death conflict that had taken place a week earlier. *Welcome home, Lisa.*

The guardian of the front door was my elderly pooch in her usual sleeping position, her hearing gone. I bent down to hug her as I scanned my home with brand new eyes. Members from church had been to the house and surprised me by tidying up and leaving enough prepared meals so I didn't have to think about nothing but resting when I first got home. I didn't know what was ahead, but I knew God would be there making a way for me.

The sinkhole that nearly swallowed me was no longer around, but the lingering trauma would tag along for the ride while I prepared to stay home on medical leave. Healing was not going to happen on its own. Like faith, it required work or it would be dead (James 2:26, NKJV). Without the watchful eyes and hand-holding from the hospital ensemble and its supporting cast, my recuperation could be in jeopardy if I didn't sustain the momentum started as an inpatient. My "ROYALTY" art piece from the hospital hung in my home as a constant reminder of my value. No booby traps or rigged setbacks would keep me from running the recovery course and riding the wave of progress to completion. I was determined to cross the finish line for a full recovery.

Little did I suspect that those traps would be laid out so soon after coming home. Navigating labor rules, which were the least kind to those impaired and unable to work from emotional abuse, was tortuous and treacherous. It was like jumping through hoops from a wheelchair. This wasn't how I expected my recuperation to begin. Each day felt like I was back at work, managing mounting projects all due at the same time. Time that should have been spent on the mend was first spent making legal inquiries, finding outpatient mental health care, creating records and submitting forms, initiating claims for medical leave and compensation, and talking to various agency staff regarding my dilemma and options.

Retelling the abuse meant reliving it. One particular occasion tested my patience with the agency's health services division, when I had to answer extensive questioning about my medical illness. The agency nurse initially challenged the length of my disability, noting it seemed like a long time to be off. In my frustration over the phone with nurse Detective Joan Friday I blurted out, "Look! He put me in the hospital!" Without skipping a beat and in perfect *Dragnet* cadence (*Just the facts, ma'am*) she retorted, "He did not put you in the hospital. You put yourself in the hospital." *Ladies and gentlemen, the story you are about to see is true. The names have been changed to protect the innocent. THE END.*

With everything I had just been through, why would a medical professional make such an ignorant comment, having no idea what the past year had been like for me? My supervisor would have sure enough killed me, had I not gotten to a hospital. The nurse's narrow thinking made me believe I had work to do in bringing awareness and sensitivity to bullying in the workplace. It's even reaching places thought impervious to intimidation, like the National Football League. As painful as it was documenting the facts that led to my mental collapse, my mind switched to autopilot to do what had to be done. Recovering would be an uphill battle, but an improvement from being down in the valley for so long.

Before recovery could officially commence, there was one small piece of unpleasant business remaining. Like condensation from a steamy shower, word must have spread by now that something had gone down. An employee who came to work every day had not been seen for weeks. Just out of the hospital, I made a gut-wrenching choice some might think was downright ludicrous. My sudden departure from work came without having a chance to remove my personal effects and private files. The coin that was launched to decide my gall or my stupidity must have been two-headed. Who would return to the place of her assault, with the assaulter still around? That was like a rape victim getting back into the bed where the rape occurred.

I emailed my manager and copied several others, including branch and division chiefs. To his chagrin, the cat had to be out of the bag. The Great Wall of Concealment was crumbling; one of his prisoners had escaped to report the horrors she suffered. This was the first time I communicated with him since he sent me to the ER. Up until this time, I used nurses and social workers as go-betweens. I was coming to clean out my desk and unbeknownst to him, I was bringing a police escort from the agency.

Management was still up to no good, exerting his power and tightening the reins to keep things low key by granting me permission to enter his lair at what would have been my usual morning report time. Not only wasn't I going to set a clock alarm for a job from which I was on leave, I certainly wasn't going to be alone with him since chances were no one else would be around so early. He tried to move me under the cloak of secrecy to keep his crime under wraps. I defiantly emailed him and told him that I would be in at 9:30 the next morning. He insinuated that I'd be distractingly interruptive to the workflow if I didn't come in much earlier, as he wished. All I was going to do was quickly empty my desk and quietly leave, while talking to no one; he just didn't want the other workers to see him squirm for what he had done, since whispers were now circulating throughout the agency.

I arrived earlier than planned, only because I was awake and decided to get it over and done with. My manager wasn't there, THANK GOD! The one employee on site looked surprised to see me and my police escort. "I've come for my things," I explained.

She led me to a box a few feet shy of the exit, conveniently positioned out of sight and away from the rest of the staff. Management had cleared my workspace and ordered colleagues to pack my belongings. Two things were missing – my Rolodex containing all my contacts, and a work binder I'd had for years. I wanted them both back.

The Rolodex was easy. My coworker returned with it from what I presumed was her desk. The binder was planted on a shelf that used to be my workspace and when I reached for it, the policeman told me without a supervisor's approval, it had to remain on that shelf. My colleague didn't have the manager's number but she had the number to his second-in-command, his protégé and a horrible manager in her own right: both of them tortured me as a pair.

After some wrangling, I was free to take my binder. When I made it back to the parking garage I thanked the police officer, lit a cigarette, flicked the match over my right shoulder to torch the job down, then drove off into the sunset never to look back again. It was still early morning, and the quietest drive I had ever taken, even with the music pumping. Now the recovery could begin.

30 *Life After Near Death*

Had my life been a play, there would have been an act entitled, "The Great Brain Robbery." Completely in bondage, my imprisoned mind was under depression's control and confined me to a place where light could not penetrate and silence was my only visitor. While sitting before the parole board of mental health professionals and asked what I'd learned from my time in the mental house, I'd reply that depression was real because no one would voluntarily give up control of their mind.

Unclick went the pause button that reset my life. I was paroled! I was free to enter into the general population to resume living again, following a near-death sentence commuted only by God.

It had been ten days since my discharge. The night before, I had the best sleep in a long time and it came without a prescription. To be dreaming again for the sake of sound sleeping was something that had been long lost to depression. For months, I had taken prescribed sleep aids that took me under without leaving a dream imprint. When I would snap awake the next morning I would only remember taking a pill the night before and nothing else--not even falling asleep. It was coerced rest that impersonated sleep.

Waking up each morning now had become a big deal. Whether it be sprinkles of sunrise mimicking day fireflies through the narrow slits of a closed venetian blind, or that one wayward bird serenading me every morning at 4:30 from the windowsill, or me lying awake in bed smiling before my feet would touch the floor and the day began. There would be no more waking up on the wrong side of the bed. I appreciated being alive and that would always be right, no matter which side of the bed.

One evening, my daughter and I walked along a popular trail that I visited every morning for solitude and quiet time with the Master. There were many more walkers in the evenings and no shortage of traded smiles and conversational joviality. Now that I had found my way out of the wilderness, it was a lot easier for me to observe the diversity of happiness in the language of people. I was sensitive to their orchestrated laughter and contagious camaraderie. It was as if my happiness antennae had been extended and adjusted to fine tune the reception of the most minuscule traces of joy, even from far away.

I needed more than the inner peace and beauty of a scenic walking trail to keep my spirits lifted. The real work of healing would depend on the outpatient treatment I would receive. Just as my psychiatric hospital admission was voluntary, so was my follow-up care, which would resume where the hospital left off. I would have never known just how hard it would be finding a psychiatrist until I actually needed one. My health plan was not always accepted but if it was taken, either new patients weren't being seen or it would be several months before an appointment would be available.

New to me were these one-stop, do-it-all behavioral health outpatient shops staffed with psychiatrists, physician assistants and nurses, psychologists, and clinical social workers--all under one roof for comprehensive psychiatric and psychotherapy care. The first one I visited made giving up my quest for treatment easy. Nothing about the place was warm or inviting; this was in stark contrast to the feel of the hospital ward. Intake for new clients would be by walk-in only on a first-come, first-served basis once a week. By the time I arrived a few minutes past opening, there was already a wait. A plastic partition separated us from them. Like my visit to the ER, I should have brought along moral support. The place gave me the heebie-jeebies and made me very uncomfortable right away. It had the mood of a free clinic in a run-down area of town, only it was located in one of the wealthiest counties in the state and richest in the country. By the time I made it to the counter and showed my hospital discharge papers, I was told I'd have to travel to a different location farther away because they had no psychiatrist onsite.

Although they were few and far between, I finally found a more accessible behavioral health care clinic that would take me. I was assigned to a therapist--a female, specifically--as the intake coordinator felt she would be a better fit since I was still reeling from the actions of a male bully. The clinic's physician assistant would manage my medications every week. So far, so good. Prior to my health crisis, having mental health care coverage was never a consideration. I skimmed over it every open enrollment season and headed straight toward vision, dental, and prescription benefits, along with whatever coverage was pertinent to women's health. Thank God for the comprehensive mental health coverage I did have. I felt for people who needed to be in mental health treatment but had no insurance.

Once I became a behavioral health patient, my insurance company was quick to respond within days of my hospital discharge. They assigned a virtual caseworker to help me stay on track with my recovery. When I asked her why she was calling me, she explained that I was labeled a risk because of my recent psychiatric diagnosis. Had it been Alcoholics Anonymous, I suppose she would have been my sponsor to help end my use of alcohol through the Twelve Steps program. She was a real person who would call to check on me and intervene, with prior permission granted, if I exuded any signs of relapse and fell off the wagon. This additional insurance benefit was wise and proactive mental health management. I was happy to garner all the support I could get.

Now that I was in treatment and had an independent caseworker checking on me, I was on task with my mental health rehab. It was also important for me to treat myself well. Self-therapy took on many forms of pampering as I became reacquainted with the simple pleasures I had missed – time outdoors, classic martial arts films by the Shaw Brothers, live jazz concerts, and nostalgic television programming like *The Beverly Hillbillies* and *Petticoat Junction* in the mornings; *The Big Valley,*

Bonanza, and The Wild West near midday; and *Sanford and Son* by evening that reminded me of family television time in my household, when coming of age in the Gwynn Oak area of Baltimore city in the seventies was all love, peace, and happiness. Gradually I was warming up to the life I had known before my mind was abducted.

Next on my list was resuming church. It had been a month since my hospitalization and initially I had reservations about attending services. Believing well-meaning saints would overwhelm me, having heard what I'd been through, I was a bit scared and unsure how I would react. Surprisingly, it was church as usual with no fuss. For the couple of saints who were privy to my nightmare from the beginning, they loved on me with strong hugs and marveled at how far I'd come and how great I looked.

It was beautiful being back in God's house again. "Touched by a Stranger" was the sermon title and before the first word was delivered, I knew this message would speak to me. The reference scripture was Mark 7:24-37, A Gentile Shows Her Faith (NKJV). A gentile woman had faith that Jesus would cast a demon spirit from her daughter. This woman refused to believe otherwise and would not give up until her daughter was restored and completely healed. When Jesus said to her, *"Let the children be filled first, for it is not good to take the children's bread and throw it to the little dogs."* The woman responded, *"Yes, Lord, yet even the little dogs under the table eat from the children's crumbs."* Her convictions would not wane, nor her blessings be denied. *"For this saying go your way; the demon has gone out of your daughter,"* said Jesus. And just like that, the woman's situation had been turned around by sincerity and faith.

My circumstance wasn't much different from that of the gentile woman. It's so easy to judge others; I've been guilty of doing this myself. Here I was, attending church a few weeks after I'd been discharged from a psychiatric hospital, when I could have been eulogized in this same church if my situation had not been turned around. Sometimes we must check our spirits and put aside our preconceived notions when we want to demean what we don't understand. I had my own thoughts on mental illness, drawn unfortunately from too much television and one unusual experience from long ago.

The first time I encountered someone with mental illness was when Judy, a new tenant, rented the apartment above mine. Things were fine until she started keeping me awake at nights. I couldn't tell if she was marching in place or running in circles, but Judy's feet never stopped moving over top of my head. I lost a lot of sleep and productivity because of her.

One evening, Judy came outside partially dressed. Her boyfriend tried unsuccessfully to get her to return to her apartment. She then started speaking with a German accent, which I found out later was one of her "personalities." I went outside to hand her my bathrobe when she stopped scuffling with her boyfriend and locked eyes on me. I stopped where I was, way short of reaching her with my robe. My mind wanted to hand it to her but my feet wouldn't

136

take another step forward. She looked at me as if I was a threat, scaring me to the point where I was ready to throw my robe at her and run back to my apartment. That's when Judy flashed her private parts at me! Her boyfriend yelled at her to stop that, and together we tried to place my robe over her. He couldn't hold her still and I gave up trying. The police arrived to manage the situation just when I was returning to my apartment. Judy was later evicted, and I never gave her another thought because it wasn't my issue. I was just happy to finally get some decent sleep again. I felt ashamed for not being more caring about my neighbor back then.

When I became a psychiatric patient, my spirit went through a tune up as I used my time in the hospital to evolve and enlighten. Not just because of the excellent care I received from health care workers, but because I got to spend time up close and personal with other patients who were no different from me, yet similarly affected by mental illness. These faces of depression were spouses, children, siblings, best friends, colleagues, parents, church members, and neighbors from any and every profession you could fathom. My spirit was humbled and I regretted being indifferent before I entered the psychiatric realm.

The strangers who touched me came by way of dedicated medical professionals. They nurtured this bewildered, scared, broken mess of a person out of a crisis and, without hesitation or judgment, cared enough to tell me I did the right thing by coming to the hospital for help. I suppose this was how the gentile woman felt. Her daughter needed help, and not healing her was not an option. The Apostle Paul said, *"do not be conformed to this world, but be transformed by the renewing of your mind, that you may prove what is that good and acceptable and perfect will of God"* (Romans 12:2, NKJV). I'd been changed for God's glory with a new mind, never to be the same again.

31 *Go with the Flow*

I had to make good use of my healing period, so I devoted my time to several unfinished community service projects I had neglected due to the job. It was freelancing without pay for causes that lifted the human spirit, and I arose early in the morning and retired late into the evening for what was a labor of love on all fronts. This was my new job for now, thinking of others and serving fresh out of the wilderness. I resumed my passion for higher learning by volunteering for my church's annual Historically Black Colleges and Universities (HBCU) College Fair. Every year I donated a complimentary scholarship resources guide that I've authored, listing hundreds of opportunities specific for underserved populations. This packet has made its way around the country and remains in high demand more than five years after our inaugural HBCU college fair.

A behind-the-scenes and out-of-sight worker, my next project involved researching fundraisers, soliciting volunteers, creating networking opportunities, and running social media for a local nonprofit organization providing temporary housing for homeless women and their children. What followed was a prematurity awareness campaign I spearheaded to share ways for educating women about premature births, which disproportionately affected the African American community.

Being in the zone meant many more projects would fill my days while I stayed home recuperating. These personal missionary assignments that reflected goodwill causes not only promoted my healing and restoration, but they also caressed and nourished my confidence until I was fit to enter the workplace again. In between the *pro bono* project management and psychiatrist and psychotherapist sessions, finding a job and having income were distant thoughts.

As if having a life-changing, near-death experience wasn't enough, I found myself grieving the loss of my four-legged companion of eleven years. I watched Duchess die unexpectedly not long after my hospital discharge. The vet had just been called after I noticed her labored breathing. Minutes later, her breathing stopped. There went my heart. Duchess died in her favorite spot, near the front door. If misery was looking for company, it wasn't hard to find at all. My canine's nuzzling, bad-breath kisses, and comedic antics got me through many gloomy days. Fiercely loyal, she stayed underfoot so much she got in my way, like when I would work on concurrent projects that were spread all over the floor in perfect order but she thought they made for good sleeping mats instead. When my daughters tried to give me a break and coax her from underneath me, they were often met with a growl, sometimes a snap and, on rare occasions, a bite. Duchess was a special needs dog with epilepsy that I had rescued from a shelter in West Virginia. She was my gift to my girls but she became the keeper of the castle, and I her mistress. Now she was gone.

Feeding the geese around the local lake whose habitat were grounds for easy mediation filled the void of not having my beloved pooch. Warnings were posted all over, telling us not to feed the wildlife, but no one paid attention to those signs. I invested in some environmentally-friendly bird food. What the geese didn't eat, the fish below them gobbled up. Recognizing the rattle of my tin canister, my newfound friends would come from all directions to eat, racing clear from the other side of the lake. However, there was always one lone goose in the distance, only watching but never joining his feasting comrades. Whenever I tried to feed it, the other geese would chase it away. I don't know what offense warranted treating a member of their own flock this way, but it was a dilemma from recent events I related to very well. My exiled friend won my compassion and all the extra morsels I kept from the others.

As news spread of what I had been through, former colleagues reached out to me with heavy hearts of disbelief. Of all the people they knew, they said, they were so sorry to hear it happened to a person like me. To be honest, I harbored those same sentiments, wondering what had I done to be the target of so much hate. It was incredibly humbling to be so well considered. Poo happens, as the saying goes for explaining the uncontrollable, unpredictable misfortunes of life. But the word of God more eloquently states in Matthew 5:45 (NKJV), *"that you may be sons of your Father in heaven; for He makes His sun rise on the evil and on the good, and sends rain on the just and on the unjust."* I was going to own my recovery and fight for possession of my mind and control over my life.

32 *Truth is Stranger Than Fiction*

While serving in the US Army Reserve as a Combat Medical Specialist, there was one activity I never looked forward to: running. I hated middle-distance running, but the physical fitness regimen always included a daily running exercise, and a timed two-mile run test you had to pass to successfully complete your training. I always ran out of steam and ended up walking some of the way. Even the few times I was fortunate enough to continue the run, I always fell behind the platoon. It never failed: before you knew it there would be the platoon, then there would be me bringing up the rear from a noticeable distance. No amount of encouragement from my fellow soldiers could help me keep running without quitting.

One morning, my first sergeant saw me lagging behind and made me report for remedial Physical Training (PT). I told him I could still pass the test, but he wasn't moved. Remedial PT was embarrassing because everyone else knew you'd failed some component of the regimen. While other soldiers had down time to chill, we remedials had to continue working out. I was really bummed about it until one day the first sergeant asked, "If I'm ever wounded on the battlefield, how do you expect to get to me to save my life?" From then on, I viewed PT differently and don't think I ever stopped to walk again. This was the proper use of perspective.

Telling a person who was receiving the blows that she was not being hit, was the wrong use of perspective. In this instance, the agency's stance that there was no evidence to support that my supervisor did anything unethical was nothing more than a weak cover-up. Something happened on the job that the agency could no longer camouflage or deny: I nearly lost my life to mental illness. It progressed from psychological molestation and ended with an all-out mental gang rape and mind execution at the hands of one of their trusted leaders.

Three months following my psychotic episode, the agency responded to the Washington, DC Navy Yard shootings with a system-wide email. I was appalled and grieved when I found out about the shootings. All the victims did was go to work on a Monday morning, with every expectation of returning home later that evening. By the next day, I wondered if the shooting involved a direct supervisor. Reports indicated the answer was no.

The email listed resources on safety and security. For a second, I couldn't read any further. I would never make light of the agency's reaction to this tragedy, but where was their concern for my safety and security when I was in the direct line of fire of an abusive manager? I learned, for the first time, that the agency had an elite team of staff in place that specialized in preventative workplace violence, as well as its aftermath. Ironically, this team was made up of representatives from some of the same offices where I initially sought help. The solution for preventing violence at work was nothing more than provisional resources that read

144

from an agency's point of view. Nothing in the resource listings supplied by the agency addressed what I had just gone through. The resources offered nothing concrete and of value for stopping a runaway, power-smug supervisor who drove workers to concerning behaviors that could lead to acts of violence at work in the first place; my "suspicious" conduct would have been considered the catalyst for this elite team to respond, and not the precursory workplace actions leading to my mental illness.

I'm being bullied by management and want to kill him! I envisioned this special elite team springing into action for this scenario, and leading me right off the premises with a restraining order in tow. Meanwhile, management would still be on the job wreaking havoc without being reprimanded. I can't be the only person bullied on the job, as many stories remain to be told. The early intervention they described for curtailing violence and maintaining employee wellbeing and productivity failed for me.

Survivors of horrendous management would make the best consultants and be the most credible witnesses for how management shouldn't be. Don't waste taxpayer dollars on task forces or oversight committees when managers start getting slaughtered by their victims. I would testify in court for the defense of any bullied employee. I'd also tell you not only what did not work, but what could have possibly prevented my depression and homicidal ideation, which were one-hundred percent manufactured from an adverse work environment I did not create!

145

Once I developed thoughts of killing and dying, the agency (whose perspective was now irrelevant) should have stopped defending their leader. I was harassed; this was the truth. Stop telling workers what they have not endured, if you are not in a position to treat or diagnose them.

33 Dr. Who

I needed to establish a medical rapport and trail to support my claim that my job had made me ill. The outpatient care treatment center I chose to help with my recovery knew from the start I was pursuing workers' compensation. The physician assistant (PA), who voluntarily gave me her cell phone number and told me she was my new BFF, assured me I would be given any supporting documentation needed for my case. Sharing high fives and hugs from behind her office door, she shared her loathing for the person who did this to me because she, too, had been in a similar situation. It seemed all was working for my good as I updated my family on the progression of my care, and never once questioned why I was under the care of a physician assistant-- rather than a psychiatrist--so soon after my hospital discharge. I just wanted to be well again, and went with the first practice that was available--after having no luck trying to make appointments with other psychiatric professionals I had reached out to. Things were moving along and coming together, or so it seemed.

I should have known something was amiss when I asked the PA for a medical letter declaring my injury for workers' compensation. She did an about-face and gave me the runaround by changing the date each time the letter was supposed to be ready. The clinic wasn't living up to my expectations; I felt my recovery was in jeopardy. So far, not so good.

With a deadline looming hours away for submitting my workers' compensation claim, the PA chose that time to inform me that their center did not do workers' compensation cases, I would not be getting a letter, and she was sorry. She hastily slapped together a copy of my medical records, most of which were the same hospital documents I'd already provided to the clinic during intake, and she handed them over to me.

My composure was astonishingly commendable, considering the ramifications of her blunder. It could have been I was just too shell-shocked and too disbelieving to react. Internally I was in agony, but managed to drive all the way home before I released all the moans and screams I had previously stifled with all office staff eyes on me.

For the second time in the past few months, I felt like dying. I trusted this clinic with my care and when I needed them the most, they failed me and torpedoed what little progress I had made into a tailspin. Even the PA's demeanor changed. I was now "ma'am" when not behind her office door, and she turned cold and brief during those encounters. She treated me like I was that one-night bad decision you never wanted brought up again. Dozens of appointments in three months, and I had nothing to show for them other than her confessed ignorance that she didn't know the clinic declined workers' compensation claims. The one time I pressed the PA to see a psychiatrist, my meeting with the doctor took less than five minutes and accomplished nothing other than discovering she knew my treating psychiatrist from the hospital. It was a legal racket. Their pockets fattened at my expense--and at the expenses of my insurance company--with every appointment that went nowhere. I left their practice, never to return.

The center's therapist phoned me days later. I explained what went down with the PA and how it adversely affected me. She then asked, what did that have to do with her? Really? For one, my therapy sessions at this clinic felt like bad first dates that time looped, replaying the same conversations over again, ending up where we started with each new appointment. I wasn't comfortable with the long pauses and stares between our exchanges, and I found myself looking more at the time and out the window, than at the therapist. It had everything to do with her, the clinic, and my stymied progress they just compromised. I thought I was going to end up back in the hospital because of how low they made me feel. Thankfully, the medication I was on must have taken effect and worked. I rebounded from this unexpected setback without lingering too long in despair.

I did what these "medical professionals" told me to do, not realizing I should have been a lot further along in my rehabilitation than I was. Had the letter fiasco not happened, I probably would have still been seeing them and gaining little progress. Those three months were not a total loss. I did get a medical disability letter early on, and that was golden. For now, I had to throw myself back into the psychiatrist-shopping market. I was still riding solo and a one-person act on this mental merry-go-round.

The next outpatient care treatment center I chose told me three months earlier that they could not see patients recently discharged from the hospital, because their facility couldn't provide the intense care a newly released psychiatric patient routinely needed. Now that three months had passed, I could be seen at this center and had an initial consultation with an actual psychiatrist, not a PA as before. It made me wonder even more why a PA had provided for my care to begin with.

On my first visit I met with Doctor Who, the mind whisperer who would be my new psychiatrist. I'm of the belief that physicians should set the bar for healthy living. If I had gone by looks alone, I may have opted for a different psychiatrist. He was a fairly large man whose size might have indicated that his health was at risk for a stroke, diabetes, high blood pressure, and heart disease--conditions which have claimed many members of my family. *How are you going to take care of my mind when it looks like your weight is not healthy?* Given my track record, I could not afford another delay to my recovery and proceeded with this new consensual relationship.

We may not have traveled through time preventing the forces of evil from hurting good people, as in the *Doctor Who* television series, but I was taken on an adventure into the world of psychiatry. One thing for sure, my new doctor was on my side to mend the destruction the evil forces (like my supervisor) had left behind.

I am certain all psychiatrists took classes on poker faces because once again, I poured out my story through an avalanche of tears and got nothing back. While I was in the middle of my depression and before I was hospitalized, I complained to every doctor I had an appointment with about the job. Whether it was the otolaryngologist, the ophthalmologist, or the dentist, I always won the doctor's sympathy, earning a hug during the exam and sometimes a prayer petition. This was never the case with anyone I encountered from the psychiatric field. Retelling my story three months later still was painfully emotional for me and when I was done, Doctor Who took me behind the scenes of mental health care, where he divulged why my care up until this point had been lacking.

He wasn't shy about expressing how psychiatrists should be better compensated for the myriad of services they provided. I learned psychiatrists were very much needed but underpaid and underappreciated, much like teachers and policemen. Many of them won't even deal with insurance companies because the sliding scale in place made them lose a lot of money. The same reasoning applied for the handling of workers' compensation claims. The massive paperwork was time-consuming and it paid poorly, dragging compensation out way too long for physicians. Using physician assistants saved money and helped a practice's bottom line prosper. Only in my case, a healthy bottom line for them forged a medical setback for me.

I appreciated all he shared, especially acknowledging that the end goal was to get me to a place independent of him and his happy pills. The previous clinic had strung me along with no end date in sight, whereas he planned to sever that string for my best interest--a relationship break up that wouldn't make me sad. My treatment was now appointments with him every six weeks supplemented with weekly therapy sessions, and it was my choice if I wanted to use an in-house therapist. He seemed ethical and prudent in doing what he was supposed to do to cure me.

He won me over after we had established that I could never return to that job. This was the first time a mental health caregiver definitively stated what I had only hoped. For the first time in three months, I exhaled. I chose a therapist from this new clinic who turned out to be a breath of fresh air. It felt like I was chatting with a longtime girlfriend over tea for an hour that always went by too fast. In our meetings she spoke candidly, sharing tidbits from her life which made it easy to talk and relate to her.

Psychiatric care would not be inexpensive, even with the best insurance. Everything became itemized and billable outside of what insurance would cover--medical letters and forms for the job and workers' compensation, medication authorizations, some consultations, and even phone calls. If, on average, you visit your primary care physician twice a year at $25 a copay per visit, do the math if you are visiting therapists and/or psychiatrists weekly for a year.

34 *Bureaucracy at Its Least Finest*

"Oh! What a tangled web we weave, when first we practice
to deceive."

Sir Walter Scott, *Marmion*

One of my favorite stories, no matter the season, is Charles Dickens' *A Christmas Carol*. Ebenezer Scrooge's redemption, and change of heart from unsympathetic to kindhearted, never grows old with me. Four spirits cared enough for Scrooge's plight to scare him straight, transforming him through eye-opening life lessons. Scrooge's only friend and business partner, Jacob Marley returned from the dead to warn his friend Ebenezer to atone for his wrongdoings in life or suffer eternal consequences later.

"'Business!' cried the Ghost, wringing its hands again. "Mankind was my business. The common welfare was my business; charity, mercy, forbearance, and benevolence, were, all, my business. The dealings of my trade were but a drop of water in the comprehensive ocean of my business!" (Charles Dickens, *A Christmas Carol*)

Mankind may not have been Scrooge's business, but it has become my business to keep what happened to me from happening to another. I may not have had the greed and selfishness of a Marley, nor bore a scythe while draped in black while forecasting the future (like the Ghost of Christmas Yet to Come), but I am the voice of experience and bring a premonition based on what occurred. A dead woman tells no tales, but I lived--for such a time as this--to tell it all.

I'd like to think that Jacob Marley's spirit finally rested in peace because of the good that came from Ebenezer Scrooge's redemption. I, thinking for the greater good just as Marley had, could never rest as long as workers were falling to bullies on the job. I would hate to see someone succeed where I'd failed with suicide, just to escape a brutish manager. But before I could advocate for downtrodden workers, I had to first advocate for myself.

Work website references for leave matters and income options were like a smorgasbord: there was some of everything, but you weren't quite sure where to start. The information on my computer screen looked like a computer programming language that needed decoding. Do I qualify or do I not qualify? Do I go this route, or another route? Can I sign up for benefits over here, and not lose benefits over there?

How nice would it have been to have all the information I needed in one place, written in plain language and streamlined into a single, concise table with seamless flow. Management was supposed to be very hands on with this process in his role as my supervisor but as you can imagine, he didn't help me with anything, nor would I have wanted his involvement. I had to connect the dots of these self-service, informational websites to decipher my best options, since no one from the agency side was guiding me.

The US Equal Employment Opportunity Commission (EEOC) was an agency known for protecting the rights of workers who'd faced discrimination (e.g., age, race, and religion) in the workplace. Employee Relations, EAP, or the ombudsman never mentioned EEOC, even after I'd said that I'd been singled out for retaliation.

Bullying didn't seem to have a place of its own among the different types of discrimination. It should have had its own large square checkbox: BULLYING. It was the ultimate form of harassment, and didn't need to have a secondary association with some of the more common types of discrimination. Bullying alone is detrimental regardless for its reasons, none of which are right.

By the time I was well enough to consider legal action, it was too late to file an EEOC complaint. It took ten months of working for my manager to develop acute mental illness and would take many more months of subsequent medical treatment to moderately recover, yet I was only given forty-five days from the first time the harassment occurred to initiate a complaint. Attorneys even offered their heartfelt sorrow (go figure) and well wishes for all I had gone through on the job, but regrettably were unable to help me.

Had the statute of limitations not run out and I had taken legal action, it was plausible I could have received a large financial settlement, easily (Tully, 2014). I ended up in a psychiatric hospital, ready to kill myself and management too! My mental illness fell short of committing a workplace massacre. That alone should have been worth a nine-figure settlement. If a law firm was looking to drum up some business, it would need to look no further than the waiting room of a psychiatrist's place of business.

It was just as well. I didn't think my fragile and injured state of mind could have withstood the challenging EEOC process. I discovered there were many steps involved before I could even file a formal complaint. From my past experiences with EAP and the ombudsman, two of those steps included words I had come to despise and no longer appreciated: counseling and mediation. No, thank you!

Now that it had hit the fan, debt was imminent as I incurred significant medical expenses from being injured on the job. I needed supplemental income from the wages I had lost while I was recovering at home. The Office of Workers' Compensation Programs (OWCP), an agency known for providing compensation to injured federal workers, was a good place to start. I now had a psychiatrist who was willing to back my claim.

It was important to show that I was in treatment for my injury so that I could validate my need for workers' compensation. I should have called on friends and family to help me sort through the bureaucratic details; it was too much for one person to tackle. I was running around completing forms, tracking deadlines, writing statements, placing phone calls, and sending emails--instead of resting and recovering like I should have been. There was very little time to rest after I left the hospital. I had a short turnaround time for reporting my injury to OWCP. The enormous amount of time and energy required to prove I had acquired a work-related mental illness revealed a new set of problems that made me feel like I was a victim all over again. Even with my PTSD diagnosis and other medical evidence, this fight would not be for the faint of heart or mind.

Once I initiated a workers' compensation claim through OWCP, I entered a world that made being a first-time mental patient in a psychiatric hospital seem like a walk in the park. The psychiatrists and attorneys I sought shunned workers' compensation cases, and I was beginning to understand why. As a psychiatric survivor of workplace abuse, I found out quickly how unfriendly OWCP was to workers impaired by psychological injuries.

That's when OWCP seemed to morph into some kind of animal that would make the beast in the Book of Revelation look like Mary Poppins. Worker was fine before starting new job; worker went insane after the job started. You would have thought my case was cut and dried, considering I never had a mental disorder before. I started to believe it was called workers' compensation because you had to work unduly hard for your rightful compensation.

As soon as I contacted OWCP with a claim of a hostile work environment--which led to psychiatric impairment--all of my contact with my manager should have ceased. His oversight of me should have been transferred to someone else in the interim when allegations of conduct unbecoming a supervisor and detrimental to work mission were levied.

Because he was still my supervisor, everything related to my disability had to be routed through him: medical updates, OWCP business, timesheets, agency forms, and leave status updates. I was in constant communication with him throughout my half-year-long medical leave of absence. The worst thing you could do to a victim was have her in contact with the perpetrator. This was deplorable, counterproductive to my healing, unfair, and plain old wrong!

Case in point: my supervisor tried to manipulate me when I needed him to sign a form that would have allowed me to receive donated leave hours--in extenuating medical circumstances--from fellow agency employees. When he read the medical statement that cited an "adverse work climate" as the cause of my illness, my manager refused to sign the form unless my doctor agreed to remove the incriminating remarks first.

OWCP was just as uncooperative and made it extremely hard for me to move my claim along. This only made for more (poop) fan-hitting target practice. This agency didn't seem to have a handle on mental disorders. OWCP was treating my mental illness like a muscle sprain, ligament tear, or broken bone--things that can be easily identified and quantified with regard to cause and recovery. The abstract and subjective rubrics OWCP relied upon for mental claims were missing the mark and failing our workers.

My mind wasn't a limb or appendage that could be reset with a cast and whipped back into shape by physical therapy. If you broke an arm, you could use the uninjured arm to compensate for the broken arm. Likewise, if you sprained an ankle, you could perform some tasks from a seated position to rest the injured ankle. Mental illness was much more complex. Healing of the mind depended on the individual's ability to discern, reason, and feel while the mind was in a vulnerable state.

Suppose that a US Postal Service (USPS) mail carrier developed a fear of dogs after being attacked by one along a mail route. USPS could make accommodations for the "psychologically-wounded" employee in a few ways. They could change the worker's route to one without dogs--like apartment buildings where dogs weren't allowed. This way, the worker could still be productive as the trauma from being bitten waned over time. If the effects from the trauma lasted a lot longer for the worker, then USPS could restrict the injured employee to duties that didn't require working outdoors. It was reasonable to believe that a postal worker could continue to work while recovering from mental trauma, in either of these two examples.

My situation was different: I was attacked by a bully and developed symptoms that were debilitating enough to be admitted to a psychiatric hospital. I was dealing with lingering negative thoughts I could only associate with pain and trauma. My "sprained" mind required rest and absence from anything related to work: my supervisor, profession, and tasks; the job, work grounds and surrounding area; my agency, field, and entire department. How then could I compensate for my psychiatric disorder, and perform modified work for the agency while I was still impaired by my illness? It wasn't possible.

A heap of hospital records meant nothing if I couldn't get a medical doctor, specifically a psychiatrist, to declare that management caused my mental illness. As God would have it, my psychiatrist was well versed in OWCP vernacular; he used to be a consultant for the agency. I was so glad to have him as my doctor. He wasn't happy with OWCP's convoluted policies either. Nevertheless, he knew exactly what to write to connect my illness to management. The medical narrative that he so eloquently crafted was a brilliant piece of writing and the more I read it, the better I felt. *Sic 'em, Doctor Who!*

During one particular visit with my psychiatrist, he asked if I wanted to apply for unemployment. I was surprised it was an option, since the agency never mentioned it. The Unemployment Insurance Program (UIP) provided short-term financial assistance to workers who were without work. I was temporarily disabled and unable to work. Since I didn't have disability insurance, UIP seemed like a sensible choice. However, I didn't know if I would have jeopardized my employee health insurance if I'd accepted unemployment benefits. My mental health care coverage under my current plan was very good. Also, both of my daughters were in college and depended on my plan.

Everyone has a right to gainful and healthy employment without being boxed and limited by what others misconstrue as being too finicky, ungrateful, and lazy, while collecting unemployment benefits. I, for one, was not going to trade one fire pit for another and had every right to take my time and choose my next employer carefully. It was better for unemployment insurance to fill in the gap of not having wages, than to work in a hostile environment whose end results were now known.

I had worked uninterrupted for nearly thirty years and was entitled to use unemployment insurance as best I saw fit. I declined to use it, however, choosing instead to continue in my leave without pay (LWOP) status. I had no doubt that OWCP would do what was right and justified--in spite of their hard-nosed business practices--when it came time to make their decision for my injury claim.

Sadly, my hopes were quickly dashed when OWCP did not do the right thing--they denied my claim. It was painful to read why my claim was not accepted. Not only was the denial letter riddled with errors and misstatements of some of the facts, it read like I was responsible for causing my own illness, just because I did not take to management's style of supervising. My PTSD was described as a self-generated emotional reaction, and OWCP referred to some of my supporting medical documents as simple excuses. Imagine that: I was to blame for ending up suicidal in a psychiatric hospital. It didn't matter that I could have died. Maybe it's more feasible to say that my tax dollars, which contributed to the federal funding of my agency and the operating expenses of my manager, put me in a mental institution.

I did not ask to be incapacitated by a bully but if there were systems in place to assist employees like me in my time of need, then why treat me the way management and the agency did, like I did not matter?

I served my country honorably, even being on standby for Desert Storm, if called. I was a law-abiding citizen who once worked up to three jobs to support my family. I worshipped faithfully, volunteered for various community and civic causes without expecting anything in return, and would gladly help anyone in need. The first time I'm injured on the job, I learned the hard way that OWCP was known as the agency that denied claims. This hurt me almost as much as the actual illness itself. OWCP left me to drown by refusing to accept my injury claim and thus, rectify the situation. I was tired of sinking! This time, I chose to swim. I filed an appeal.

35 *When Your Mind is Raped by a Bully*

And I saw the beast, and the kings of the earth, and their armies,
gathered together to make war against him that sat on the horse,
and against his army. And the beast was taken, and with him the
false prophet that wrought miracles before him, with which he
deceived them that had received the mark of the beast, and them
that worshipped his image. These both were cast alive into a lake
of fire burning with brimstone. And the remnant were slain with
the sword of him that sat upon the horse, which sword proceeded
out of his mouth: and all the fowls were filled with their flesh.
Revelation 19:19-21 (KJV)

I've been through enough legalese within my agency and
outside of my agency to know that justice delayed is justice denied.
A supervisor who was responsible for my mental illness still has
his government job, and this is not justice. I've got an inferno
living inside my gut because of the damage caused from his
psychopathic agenda. If hurting people hurt people, then my goal
is to kill my enemy with these words: You are a mental rapist!

Unconsented sex by force, is the first thing that comes to
mind when you think of the word "rape." Rape has also been used
to describe "an act of plunder, violent seizure, or abuse."
(Dictionary.com) My mind was raped by a bully on the job. I
don't remember my transition to crazy, only that I had arrived

there. I reverted back to a child, wishing I had my mommy. She called out to me once, and startled me from my sleep. "Lisa!" she yelled. I lifted my head off the pillow and strained my eyes to see in the darkness. "Yes?" I replied, while looking in the direction from which my mother's voice came. Then I realized it was just a dream. Or was it?

What I wish had only been a dream was a part of my life that had been stolen from me. Imagine that I've awakened from a depression stupor, disoriented and in shock, not knowing exactly where I was but suddenly realizing how I got there. My thoughts were mine again, once I had wrestled them from up under depression's control. Outrage was the only connector to my right frame of mind, which up until this point had been docked in the wrong frame from psychological abuse. May the following letter I've written to my enemy be the conduit for purging my soul of anger, and freeing my will for total peace.

Dear Management:

Had I taken my life, I know you wouldn't have had any remorse. My thoughts for what I'd like to have happen to you were savage. Savagery may be your way of thinking, but it is not mine. I was like a goose, happily gliding along in anticipation of that next exciting adventure. Then I came to work for you.

Scripture from the New Testament, Revelation 19:17-21 describes the defeat of God's enemies. They were burned alive, the rest killed by sword--their carcasses were fed to the fowls. In the end, none of the wicked survived. That is what I'd like to see happen to bullies like you. I want these enemies of the workplace to be eradicated. You tried to destroy this wondering, carefree spirit but now that my wounds have healed, it will be happy feasting. Only, it won't be fowls gorging themselves on dead flesh; it will be the feasting of a you-reap-what-you-sow payback known as karma, instead. And it is going to cook your goose!

The people in your circle must think you're quite the phenom. The people in my circle think you're a phenomenal piece of work, an extreme mental case. You were just like the Dr. Jekyll/Mr. Hyde character in Robert Louis Stevenson's novel. You knew when to turn on your best face for your associates, then flip to reveal the bad side of you when no one was watching. After I fell for your ploy that I'd be working in a great environment, I found out there was never a good side to you; I always saw the monster.

You think you can play God, be a fate master, and destroy good-natured souls at will for sport and hobby? Scripture says to turn the other cheek (Matthew 5:38-41)--I'm supposed to offer you my remaining cheek to pimp slap while resisting the urge to retaliate. What I look like, handing you a second go at trying to kill me?

I don't think so! You were Satan's top choice for Operation Annihilate Lisa, but you didn't count on me surviving. I survived to rat out asinine managers like you from the workplace. Your mind-plundering days are over! Who's your bully now?

I don't know if I'm angrier because you're male or because you're African American. Chivalry was dead, and you were a discredit to your people. From young, gifted, and Black to just plain ole dumb and sick! Let's call a spade a spade; you ruined the Black professional persona as only you could. You were supposed to pay it forward and lend a helping hand to those coming behind you. After you made it, you made sure that others did not.

Were your ancestors preserved in a time capsule during slavery in America, and impervious to centuries of oppressive conditions? Based on your habitual cruelty, did you even know slavery ended? Shamefully and proudly, Maryland housed the two most famous slaves turned freedom fighters: Harriet Tubman (who was also known as "Black Moses") and Frederick Douglass. Both of them fought to free the ones who were coming behind them. I wonder if our Black Moses would have left your ancestors behind on the Underground Railroad, had she known your lineage would produce a modern-day slave master. Fifty years post boycotts, sit-ins, and marches did not give you the right to use your academic pedigree to be an Oreo lyncher of your own kind.

Your position was not a license to gut honest workers and hang them out to rot. You and I stand on the shoulders and backs of legends, giants, and martyrs whose fights--and even deaths--helped us both get to where we are today. I don't know if I would have had the courage to fight beside them had I come along then, but the least I can do now is protect what they fought and died for. I owe them that, and so do you!

Harboring so much anger is not healthy and I want to move on and forgive you, though not easy. You may never face prosecution for what you did to me, and I should be upset about that, but what the judicial eternal process down below has in store for you will be punishment enough. I was angry-mad and mad-crazy enough to want to kill you. Do you understand that you almost died? You drove me there! But you had help from an agency that should have grown a pair and castrated your ego trip to stop your predatory assault on employees, and to keep you from cranking out more monster managers under your tutelage.

The effects of bullying went beyond harming just me. When you messed with me, you messed with my family and as anyone knows, a mother bear in the wild will decapitate anyone who's perceived as a threat to her cubs. Your assault on me would have continued until the day my daughters became motherless. Just the thought of this makes me boiling mad! Yeah, so the chip on my shoulder is a muthalovin' boulder right about now. Who could blame me?

It would be interesting to see if you would survive public opinion. In a just world, you would be found guilty of being unfit to manage workers, lose your job, and go to jail for cruel and unusual punishment against man. Certainly, you should go to trial for assault with the intent to force a death by suicide. You're a criminal and deserve getting the work over in prison that you dished to me. May your jail friendships be everlasting. There, I hope that karma will be ten times the friend to you than depression was to me. A punk bully you is, but a gansta you ain't.

"DEAD! From an overdose of hate," might have read my tombstone. I believed in the goodness of people until I met you. You are a sadist and I did everything I could to perform my duties under your tyranny and brutality. Actually, I was incredibly brilliant to have held my own as long as I did before caving. I did it for the people depending on the projects and I felt bad for them, because they had no idea a lunatic was at the other end of the pipeline delivering calamity and mayhem. If my life ever depended on one of your projects, I would reject it for a different option because chances are, you destroyed human beings achieving your own self-serving agenda.

If an animal was sick beyond cure, it would be put down to end its suffering. Do you think you should be put down, to end the suffering of others? You preferred chaos and destruction to professional and civility. My name, my integrity, and my character meant a lot to me and I defended them in truth and honor, which meant publically exposing you as a fraud. My punishment would be a wrath more destructive than a tsunami.

Managers like you done bougie-rized Black-on-Black crime. I even delayed reporting you--dealing with your nonsense--because I thought about the many outstanding African American professionals coming behind you, who might not get a chance to blaze the trails you've single-handedly managed to destroy with your fall from grace. Profiling doesn't just happen on America's streets, it happens in the work place too.

You've done nothing but squash people on your way up, leaving causalities all along the way after you used workers for what you wanted and drained the life out of them. You mastered misery and strife at the intersection of lunacy and narcissism but, in all your educational brilliance, you had no clue how to be a decent human being and set a shining example for future leaders--and that's just tragic. No, that's just dumb!

No one acts this psycho unless they are guarding something. Rumors were always rampant that you'd had inappropriate relationships, enticing prospective conquests with chilled wine through an ambience of scented candles from behind your office door. Did I jinx your mojo? Was I a threat to your lust smuggling? I nearly died because of your thirsty appetite for vanilla latte and green tea skirts!? We will never know unless someone has the wherewithal to investigate you (watch those emails start getting deleted).

I wonder how different things would have been had I killed the root of all evil. The agency would have been lightning fast to respond, instead of giving the wussy runaround as they'd done to me. The country's leaders would have demanded to know how a little not-so-old lady from church was driven to kill her boss. It would have been reactive medicine, like everything else, waiting for something to first go wrong when there should have been proactive, preventative planning all along.

The writing was clearly on the wall that a sniper hit was coming on a rogue who was dropping employees like flies. If I had killed you and lived to be a character witness for workplace injustice, would I have had the sympathy of an unhappy working class who can relate to what I'd been through: the hate of all unscrupulous management who will now have oversight and diminished power? Or would I be the reason behind responsible legislation that would swiftly denounce and remove managers who create unsafe and unhealthy work cultures?

Even if all I've just said ever made it before a court of law as my victim impact statement, it would be hard for me to gloat over your pending doom. I have every right to be angry but even in my rage, I can't wish what I went through on another human being. I have an obligation to forgive and I'm working on it, but for now I can't help but pity you because obviously you have no idea what it means to have real joy. Ironically, because of the wilderness you created for me, I do. No job is worth death. Maybe you were bullied as a child for being a Black nerd and just went boo coo crazy for revenge when you got some power. This is not an excuse to be inhumane! Rather, this should have been the reason for you to lead with a passionate rapport.

I survived and took flight to help other wounded flocks fly again. If I should see you today, I don't know what my reaction would be. My mind can't dissect evil but it can condense you to a nightmare that ceases to exist. *Poof! Be gone with you!* You're dead to me. Where there was rage, I now feel peace.

Signed,
The Mind of a Survivor

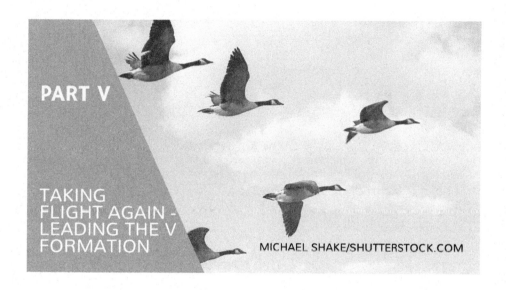

PART V

TAKING FLIGHT AGAIN - LEADING THE V FORMATION

MICHAEL SHAKE/SHUTTERSTOCK.COM

36 *Recovering a Lost Mind*

Fear not, for I am with you; Be not dismayed, for I am your God.
I will strengthen you, Yes, I will help you, I will uphold you with
My righteous right hand. Behold, all those who were incensed
against you Shall be ashamed and disgraced; They shall be as
nothing, And those who strive with you shall perish.
You shall seek them and not find them—Those who contended with
you. Those who war against you Shall be as nothing, As a
nonexistent thing. For I, the Lord your God, will hold your right
hand, Saying to you, Fear not, I will help you.
Isaiah 41:10-13 (NKJV)

Dear Management:

I am a person, and I MATTERED! Managing is not a position to maim or kill. I wish no harm on you, only for you to stop harming others. Your work mission was to enhance health and life, yet you were a health detriment to your own employees. Who would have thought a false performance evaluation was the beginning of my end? How many more workers are unfairly and negatively impacted by these power torture principles by managers like you? I'm upset you didn't value my life and more enraged that you are still on the job, lying in wait for more innocent victims. Get some help!

My help comes from the Lord, when I remember all God had done for me. You must have thought you were King Nebuchadnezzar from the Old Testament. When I did not fall down to honor your idolatrous thinking, you threw me into the fiery furnace--never counting on me having God's covering and a flame-retardant faith. With everything else that tried to destroy me, this too shall pass. A new life emerged from a near death. If it wasn't for this turbulent road you paved for me, I would have never arrived at the crossroads of bliss and peace with this unconditional love for life. A prolonged medical leave of absence from being beat down by your meanness turned out to be a lengthy and lovely peace retreat and restoration conference for a party of one. True happiness comes in the littlest of things that are often taken for granted, the least of which is simply waking up.

Thank you for doing in a few months what I couldn't do in over twenty years: lose weight and an entire size. The stress of working for you spoiled my appetite and before I knew it, I needed to treat myself to a whole new wardrobe. The truth is, I should be a little mad at joy right now. As I started to fall in love with life again and my joy returned, so did those lost pounds.

Because you seemed to think my private life revolved around you--what with all the extra work you assigned that found its way into my home every evening--I was forced to give up my salon appointments. But baby, what I stepped into was my raw essence when I embraced my silver wisdom and natural coils, and never looked back. I love the transition and thank you for helping me discover my natural outer beauty. How ya like me now?

Friends, family, acquaintances, even people I hadn't seen for some time, would greet me with a captivating curiosity, sensing something very different about me. It was a subtle observation, before I could return a greeting or exchange a smile. Whatever it was, they seemed in awe when they looked in my face, not knowing the hell you had put me through beforehand. Some would have considered it "the glow" associated with being in love, or in the family way. I was told whatever I was doing to keep doing it because I looked amazing, youthful even. It was an aura that leaked God was here, and there was nothing subtle about it. I was loving me, and life.

Those unexpected affirmations helped nurse a wounded spirit back to abundant living and overflow. You showered me with your unwavering demented devotion and all of your evil intentions, ripping me apart with your sweet nothings of my worthlessness and insignificance. That malarkey had me ready to embark on a one-way trip, with depression leading the way. Thank you, enemy, for making my inner beauty shine brightly.

For a season, I thought my name was "unacceptable" and "unsatisfactory," your daily salutations to me in endless emails since you rarely spoke to me. You may never change, but I'm in too great a place now to care if you would ever apologize for nearly killing me. I changed and for that, I thank you. Repent for all the wrongs you've done, before it's too late. Instead of Charles Dickens sending Christmas spirits to persuade your heart, may you receive a visit from the Holy Ghost. Boo! Having a bad day on earth is nothing like having a bad eternity.

You knew right from wrong, but you made a choice to do more harm than good. As a leading minority in a majority profession, others should want to emulate you. We're one generation removed from Jim Crow – we cut our teeth on its final years. People of all races made sacrifices so we could have these equal opportunities we have now. You are an example of how not to manage, rather than a model for aspiring leaders.

Over my career, I've had some amazing supervisors – ones who shut down work to allow my colleagues to pay their respects at my parents' funerals without charging time off to anyone; ones who covered my pay without asking until the furlough ended and I was able to pay them back; ones who helped me with food and clothes when times were very lean; and even those who told me it was very reasonable, and perfectly okay, to take a day off to watch the funeral of Coretta Scott King on television. I once told a supervisor that if she ever left I would follow her, even if it meant this Marylander had to relocate to Alaska. She was humbled. These were examples of respectable leaders. They had devoted followers and led with care in their hearts, not by instilling fear in our minds.

I shudder to think of all I would have missed, had I chosen death over life. One of the first things was a request to consider joining the Board of Trustees at my church. Four months prior, I was in the hospital fighting to live and now, I am trusted enough to handle one of the most important functions of the church. Not knowing what I had been through, my fellow church members saw God's best in me after I had been at my worst.

Thank God, I lived to see both of my daughters graduate from college a year later. Had they lost me, I know it would have affected their studies and derailed the educational hopes and dreams my ancestors and I had for them. You have a family, so I can only believe that you'd want the best for your children as well.

There were many more milestones and special occasions I would have missed, like my 30-year high school reunion and me celebrating the half-century mark of life with a virgin sunrise voyage in a hot air balloon overlooking the Rio Grande. I accepted your position to groom my skill set; I planned on staying until I retired. Leaving what was comfortable to step out of the box and onto a psychiatric ward was not the growth I had planned. I'm still highly sought after to lend my time, talents, and treasures for many passionate causes but of all the things I've had happen since determining to live this abundant life you tried to snuff out, having gotten the attention of a certain gentleman for an unforgettable season has got to be near the top. He knew my worth when we were adolescents and had no idea how much you hated me, and what it nearly cost him.

"I was once in love with you and that is something that I do not do (LOVE) often. I mean, what is there to not adore, cherish, protect, and love about Lisa? Unless you have forgotten your own net worth, this is something that you should expect from men like me all the time. You have class, beauty, and brains...the ultimate trifecta. You were married to a punk-ass

brother who knew that you did not have a single man in your circle to protect you. Men like him will never stand up to a real man like me. I could have protected you, as any real friend should have. I am an Entrepreneur and CEO of my own non-profit corporation; a very, very busy man. I would like to be an asset to your life, period because I know that you are worth my time....my love..... "

One of the most valuable lessons I learned while in outpatient therapy came when the world lost Nelson Mandela. I was waiting to see my psychiatrist when a patient directly across from me looked up and broke the sterility of the waiting room with, "Nelson Mandela was a great man. I don't know if I could be as forgiving." I'm not sure if his comment was directed at me, or if he was just talking out loud. I wondered if it was because I was the only Black patient in the room that he felt compelled to say that. He was Jewish. It didn't matter why he said it or who said it, because I agreed with him.

I had just seen the movie *Mandela: Long Walk to Freedom* and one of the many poignant scenes I remember from the movie came when Mandela chose to forgive, after spending twenty-seven years in captivity. Prisons aren't always confining physical structures. If he didn't forgive his jailers, then he would still be in jail. There is no place for anger and resentment for a man who wants to be really free. You may have held my mind captive, enemy, but God guarded my heart--a heart large enough to reciprocate love, but with no room to foster hate. I was grateful for this gentle reminder from a fellow patient who shared his grief over the death of Mr. Mandela. *Shalom.*

Truth will always win, and I abided in it from the moment you told the first lie on me. Proverbs 21:21 (NKJV) says, *"He who follows righteousness and mercy Finds life, righteousness, and honor."* Your downfall was your greed for evil, so eager to do me dirty that you made mistakes, which I happily exploited.

I wouldn't be able to appreciate all I have been blessed with now, thanks to His amazing grace, had it not been for all the bad I had to first go through, thanks to you. I saw the goodness in people again. New friendships would emerge along the way. Too many wonderful things have happened to me since then not to forgive you, including leaving an imprint for the world through writing. Thank you, enemy. A testimony and an example of what can go wrong but can also go right at the same time, I'm using what I have learned to advocate and be in a place where God can use me to improve the lives of those who may have been lost or wounded. Those gifts developed from adversity--and refined by Him--have made me a better human being. Not perfect, but better.

Signed,
The Heart of a Forgiver

37 *Surviving for a Testimony Such as This*

"Faith is taking the first step, even when you don't see the whole staircase."

Martin Luther King, Jr.

When I was young, and before seatbelts were required, my family and a few neighbors would cram on top of another inside my parents' Buick, and head off into the wee hours of an early Saturday morning. We'd stop for night crawlers and bloodworms at a bait and tackle shop before boarding the boat waiting to take us on a fishing excursion of Deal Island, on Maryland's Eastern Shore.

I'm not much of a fish eater today, but I have fond memories of going fishing and having fun with my cousins. It was a way of life for families who lived in the city but came from the country. Why a Chinese food-type box full of live, crawling worms didn't creep an eight year-old girl out is beyond me, but I could handle a worm and bait a hook with the best of them. All I knew was once my baited line hit the water, I could expect a fish tug at any moment and my dinner later that evening. That is, unless I reeled in a hideous-looking monster known as the toadfish.

My daddy would take it off my hook, stab it in the head with his knife, and throw it back in the water. He wasn't the only one. If a toadfish latched on to your hook it met the same fate, no matter the fisherman or child, because it was considered a pest. I can't remember if I was disturbed by the seeming brutality of this ritual, but what I can remember is how legendarily ugly this fish was, with features that would frighten away the boogeyman. It eats just about anything, when it eats at all, and thrives in poor conditions, not bothered by pollutants or litter. It can even live out of water for long periods of time. In spite of its unappealing attributes, it was those very traits that made the toadfish an important research model for metabolic studies and human balance disorders, among other things. What some fishermen considered worthless, researchers saw as having value and meaning. This is just how God works. All creatures are important to Him. He uses the least likely, according to His plan (1 Corinthians 1:28). In this instance, it was an ugly toadfish.

I'm no toadfish, but it took me crashing to rock bottom in order to gain a whole new appreciation for what God has done for me. My eyes saw through new lenses, my heart pulsed to a different beat, and my empathy for victims of bullying spearheaded a personal crusade I know was God-given and -driven. It wasn't by accident that I've become the sacrificial lamb for an assignment that isn't popular: openly discussing mental illness as an African American, in the hopes I will soften the stigma, encourage early treatment, and save a life.

I'm often asked why I didn't resign. Practically, I wasn't in a position to do so, even with the horrific abuse and no other job offers. Every promising job devastatingly fell through. I was the only means of support for two children in college, and did what I think many parents might have done. My role was to be the shock absorber, protecting and shielding my children from the bumpy, ugly dealings of life. They didn't know what the job was doing to me because I chose not to distract them with my work burdens. My daughters were almost finished with school and as their mom, I wanted nothing to deter them from fulfilling this dream.

Having survived the ordeal, I also believe resigning then, with or without a new job, would have diluted my testimony. Defeating the enemy was a mega victory! I prayed for a door to a new job to open, before I lost it. What God gave me was a new work assignment, after I had already lost it; its fringe benefits included a promotion in faith, love, and goodwill. A winning Powerball lottery ticket couldn't have matched the riches and rewards--humility, growth, and wisdom--that I achieved from one solitary bad season.

I may have taken a leap of faith, but I landed squarely into a purpose and destiny that was beyond anything I could have ever imagined for myself. I was to be a blessing in the unknown, unfamiliar, and truthfully uncomfortable as a result of a wilderness that nearly killed me.

In the end, I had to be extremely sick to consider death over my children. Depression, a nondiscriminatory and often unpredictable condition, made me afraid to live. I barely survived bullying but now understood how victims of bullying, particularly adolescent victims, welcomed death as a bully repellent. My heart goes out to their survivors. I'm proof that bullying isn't just a problem among children.

The number one question I'm asked is, what happened to my supervisor? The answer has been the same: nothing. Each door of justice I pursued was slammed shut in my face and in the faces of victims coming behind me. *Knock, knock!* Put the latch across the door if you must, but at least crack it open to see who's there. It's the voices interrupted and nearly silenced that are begging for action now, for safer work environments. Please open the door and listen to what we have to say, and then do something!

I've come across too many people who have endured some type of abuse on the job, albeit no one I know had become a patient in a mental institution. I survived what no person earning a respectable living should ever go through, and I cannot keep quiet while others are still held captive by work-induced depression from leaders who are bullies. I want to be an agent of hope and a conscience for supporting legislation that does not condone bullying in the workplace.

I had been preparing for such a time as this all of my saved life. The faith test was given when I least expected, to see if I would apply all I had been taught and learned. I didn't even try to finish the test. I gave up, turned in my paper, and completely let go to concede to death. What was the point of going on? My faith was temporarily homeless, evicted by depression. That's exactly when God stepped in. That's worth a couple of hallelujahs and several Amens! John Ogden Sr., CEO/Chairman of the Board of

Directors for the Christian Motorcyclists Association, speaks on faith or fear like this:

"Faith is shown when we lay hold of the things of God in the face of the naysayers of this world, continually pushing forward. Faith causes us to believe the best about other people. Faith causes us to look into hopeless situations and see the hand of God. Faith causes us to go the extra mile. Faith causes us to put our arms around a brother or sister that is hurting and encourage them. Faith causes us to reach out to people who have hurt or offended us. Faith causes us to love the unlovable. Faith causes us to keep going. Faith propels us towards the calling of God. Faith causes us to be strong in Him. Faith is what will mold us and make us into the image of God. Faith drives fear away. Faith brings victory and peace. To operate in faith, we must stand and follow God in the face of all obstacles for faith will allow us to see the victory when no one else can see it. Faith literally allows us to be formed into the anointed and powerful Christians that we are called to be. We are not moved by what we see or by what we feel, but we are moved by what God says. Our destiny is defined in God's Word and set forth by His blood that ran down the cross." (Ogden, Sr., 2013)

As unlikely and unorthodox as it sounds, my refuge from the enemy was an asylum, a psychiatric hospital where I received my calling to be a champion for workers' rights. I had known God for some time but it wasn't until this experience that I got to *know* Him. He's gifted me with a riveting testimony that will allow me to offer hope and encouragement to others wounded in their spirits by similar situations.

I was very optimistic about the future. It had been nearly six months since that fateful morning when I debated if I should die or not. I was still in leave without pay status from the job, and my rainy day funds were becoming arid. I was forced to make every penny count. One afternoon, I went to the Vitamin Shoppe to buy a generic brand of vitamin D supplements. There was a woman at the counter preparing to buy a case of a specialty supplement. She was trembling as if she had Parkinson's disease and the salesperson was using a calculator to give her an estimate. I figured if she was asking for the total before he finalized the transaction, then the purchase must be a financial hardship. If I had been working, I wouldn't have hesitated to step up and pay for her items. But the tugging of my heartstrings plucked my conscience and I decided to pay for her purchase anyway. It was expensive, and amounted to the equivalent of what I would have paid for a week's worth of groceries. My generic purchase was less than five dollars.

When the woman found out I was picking up her tab, she fought me tooth and nail. She wanted to know why and I answered, "Because God told me to." She asked for my name, but I wouldn't tell her. She countered with an inquiry about where I worked, and I told her I didn't.

With that, I bolted from the store in tears because I wasn't sure I did the right thing. If God was telling me to do this, then why was this woman doubting my generosity and resisting my freewill offering? I told God if she didn't want to receive my random act of kindness, then oh, well. My family needed food, my medical bills were escalating, and I didn't have the kind of duckets like that to throw away on a stranger, who told me over and over again it wasn't necessary to spend my money on her. This happened on a Monday.

Exactly one week later, on the following Monday, I was offered and accepted a job I had interviewed for weeks earlier. Maybe the woman in the vitamin store didn't need my financial assistance, but I think I did the right thing by being obedient to God's prompting. This is how I now feel about accepting a position a year earlier that initially had me leery, which turned out to be an inverted tragedy and the biggest testimony of my life. My hesitation was tabled as I obeyed the Heavenly Commander in Chief on this very special assignment. As for my resignation and twenty-four year career abruptly coming to an end, the agency thanked me for my service in a one-line statement heading my separation packet. *Goodbye and good riddance*!

If it weren't for the pain in cahoots with life's unexpected troubles, joy would be lonely and taken for granted. A faith journey I never saw coming veered into a mental health stint, which made me double-stereotyped. First, as a single African American parent; and second, as a mental health patient.

Statistically my family was doomed, labeled a broken family whose chances of succumbing to Baltimore's urban plight were highly likely. This path of solo parenting was not planned, and it wasn't pretty. I worked nonstop to make ends meet, and I was unable to take a decent vacation because I could never save for one. Many years later, my hard work paid off. I'm happy to say that my daughters graduated from the University of Maryland Eastern Shore within six months of one another, both earning scholarships and graduating debt-free, with full-time jobs in their fields awaiting them immediately post-graduation. My God provided when I couldn't. He will do no less for you.

I gave up what was comfortable and went through a painful transition. Something good has come of it: another notch in my testimonial belt for all the things I can do through Christ, who strengthens me (Philippians 4:13). It started with leaving my comfort zone and continued with my trust in Him. If I had not done what I feared, I would not have been able to share this testimony. That fear was then, my trust is now, and the end was the beginning of a new faith walk, and being in a place of total dependence on God. I love more, understand better, forgive easier, and appreciate the smallest of things.

Rejoice in the Lord always. Again I will say, rejoice! Let your gentleness be known to all men. The Lord is at hand. Be anxious for nothing, but in everything by prayer and supplication, with thanksgiving, let your requests be made known to God; and the peace of God, which surpasses all understanding, will guard your hearts and minds through Christ Jesus.

Philippians 4:4-7 (NKJV)

38 *Transcending Peace*

How do you renew a mind that was lost? It begins by appreciating the good that came from a bad situation, and syncing it to your heart. God wrapped His everlasting arms around me and held me, just when I was ready to let go and drown in the midst of a raging storm. Before, I couldn't feel God at all; now I felt Him all over me. I thanked Him for the sunshine He sent each morning to softly illuminate Billie Holiday poised over a microphone, giving me a one-on-one concert from her portrait on my bedroom's east wall. My good mornings had no more heartaches because I had finally achieved the peace I'd hoped. It was the dawning of a new day. My new lease on life equated to abundant living, which had nothing to do with the things of this world. I was rich in spirit, and that's priceless!

The outpouring of support I received as an inpatient, and since my discharge, had been nothing short of phenomenal. So many people were vital to my recovery; I can't thank them all enough. They came from near and far to offer their devotion and kindness, which helped me reach the level of peace that I enjoy today. Peace made it possible for me to go without income for months, yet not panic. If I didn't learn anything else from this experience, I learned that God pours out His blessings from the most unusual containers.

I wanted to work again, but I was also convinced that it was time for a pivotal midcareer move. I had grown weary of my field long before I launched out into the deep of this tidal-wave experience. A former colleague of mine was vacating his position at another company to move across the country. Beth, the friend I used to work with who visited me in the hospital, wanted me to consider the position. Even my psychiatrist thought it would be good for me, but it was a job similar to what I had done before and I wanted no part of it--not now, not ever!

I was still suffering from the effects of PTSD. It was perfectly understandable to bury anything remotely related to what I had been delivered from. Never mind that there were no jobs lined up, and I had been without income for months. I expected God to do a new thing in my life and I did not believe He would want me in a similar occupation that could evoke bad memories and further stress. That was not the delivery I wanted, and I refused to be overruled. The beating I took from my job left me with no confidence to continue in a field I could only associate with pain and near death. I deserved to be happy in my work after all I had gone through.

I reluctantly inquired about this position anyway, since it was practically served to me on a silver platter. The problem was that I had no appetite from the last job that was handed to me. But I also knew I could not live much longer on peace alone. I put my ex-associate in the hot seat, and I grilled him as if he was testifying before the United States Congress for a major hearing. At the end of my interrogation, I asked this: "How is your boss? Is she nice to work for?" Without hesitation, he told me that she was the best. This was the job which, as you read in the prior chapter, turned into an offer. Coincidentally, I started this new job right after OWCP had denied my claim. God's timing couldn't have been better. Today, I couldn't be any happier in what is still a great fit, all this while later.

It took real courage and the biggest faith leap to leave an agency after twenty-plus years for a new job, and in a different industry. Only God, in His infinite wisdom, power, and glory, could take a job that nearly destroyed me and have it to where the same kind of work made me utterly happy and fulfilled. Good, sound leadership who advocated for the workers and got in the trenches with us made all the difference. These leaders were very open, honest, and transparent. They invested in everything from our morale, to our potential to rise. We were appreciated, and they showed it. We mattered! No wonder this company was known for being one of the best places to work in our area. The guardian angels of quality work-life must have finally heard me. The retirement police would have to come and arrest me before I'd leave.

Here's the kicker: the job pays significantly less. However, I wouldn't trade happiness and peace for any dollar amount. I even returned to doing something I hadn't done in nearly fifteen years: I shared my career with elementary school children, and I did so with all the enthusiasm of a National Cherry Blossom Festival reveler awaiting peak blooms following a brutal and paralyzing Washington, DC winter. I must have been very convincing, because the students and staff wanted me to come back for their next Career Day.

Superficial or deep, scars from wounds need not be permanent. Once lost and mentally bankrupt, this was not just a new day, but also a beautiful life and a wonderful world--my new motto thanks to the timeless classic of the same name, as sung by Louis Armstrong. To all the members of my flock who helped and protected me while my flight was interrupted, and who made my world wonderful again, thank you and God bless you. I lived to fly again. *Welcome back, Lisa.*

39 *Don't Stand Down, Stand Tall*

I watched what I thought was going to be a nasty blood battle unfold. Sneakier than a thief in the night, I saw a heron slowly stalking a goose and her goslings as they treaded water on the edge of the pond. The pond was usually full of geese, but on this quiet afternoon it was all but deserted. Except for the tiny flock that was comfortably feeding under a soft wind, there was one lonely bird that was on the prowl for food. The first time I spotted a heron on the pond was the first time I had ever seen one. I almost didn't notice him because he stood for minutes on end without moving. Always coordinating his daily visits to the pond with my lunchtime walks, he stealthily patrolled the pond's perimeter, tiptoeing before his head vanished under water to sneak attack some prey.

There he stood still, staring at the unsuspecting family of geese from his perched position on the grass. Like a chameleon, he blended with the forest backdrop as if he was using an invisible cloak to be inconspicuous, only he wasn't invisible. The pond was large with a sprouting fountain in the middle, and it was home to many types of wildlife. When flocks of geese occupied the pond, the heron always kept his distance. He stayed far away on the other side of the pond to remain obscure while he gobbled up fish and pond vegetation. This time it was different: the heron was so close to the mom and her goslings that it was no secret he had geese on his mind for lunch.

The heron left his post and inched closer toward the pond. In real-time slow motion he lifted his long, knock-kneed legs, putting one in front of the other until he was a step away from the pond. Even with him closing in, the goose continued grazing with her goslings as though the heron didn't exist; his invisible cloak must have been working.

Whoa! The heron made a bold move that placed him in pouncing distance. He had entered the water. At this point I was supposed to look away, knowing a gosling was about to get snatched, but found myself looking on anyway out of curiosity. Then it happened.

The heron took one step too many for the goose's comfort. She turned from her grazing to square off with her challenger. She extended her neck to its full height, showed off her four-foot wingspan, and charged the heron with the speed of a roadrunner, sending him clumsily fleeing into the air. Satisfied that the threat was gone, the goose returned to grazing, like nothing happened. The heron was more than twice the size of the goose, with legs that could easily overtake an opponent; who would have ever taken the heron for a punk bird? Moreover, who would have thought that a mother goose had that much fight in her? The goose stood her ground for her cause, which was the safety of those coming behind her.

I remember watching the movie *Something to Live for: The Alison Gertz Story,* starring Molly Ringwald, when it debuted on network television in the early 1990s. Based on real events in the life of Ms. Gertz, the story portrayed a young, beautiful, and privileged female who broke the perception of what AIDS (acquired immunodeficiency syndrome) was supposed to look like. A one-night stand led to her contracting AIDS. This movie, along with the news that tennis champion Arthur Ashe had AIDS and basketball player Earvin "Magic" Johnson Jr. was positive for the human immunodeficiency virus (HIV) that caused AIDS, were the catalysts for me to view AIDS differently, as this affliction wasn't just a problem of homosexual men or needle sharers. Ms. Gertz, Mr. Ashe, Mr. Johnson, and so many others rose above the devastating diagnosis to educate the public about the disease and inspire anyone who would be similarly affected by its grim prognosis. This was nearly twenty-five years ago. I'm sure many people are alive and well today because they listened to these courageous stories from advocates who thought more about those who were coming behind them, than about the consequences of being stigmatized themselves.

I come from a culture where suicides are rarely noted. My lifestyle and health history were not risks for acquiring mental illness. If it could happen to me, then it could happen to you. Maybe because I don't appear to be what you'd expect a mental patient to be, I'll capture the public's attention and lend credence to the issue of bullying and its effects as something that not only plagues juveniles, but mature adults as well.

A group of my peers met for dinner to pay homage to a brilliant woman with a heart of gold, abundantly compassionate as she was smart. Beth accepted a new job a thousand miles away, and we gathered to say farewell and good luck to our friend. She was the first in my flock to leave the formation and render aid upon my distress while I lay grounded and unable to fly. She visited me in the hospital, rallied support from former coworkers, and helped me land a new job. Beth was the epitome of kindheartedness. If everyone had a friend like her, then there shouldn't be any mean people in the world.

When the dinner ended I worked my way around the room to mingle with the other dinner guests I had not seen for some time. We used to work happily together at one of my former jobs, before I left to go work in the hell trap I had only recently escaped. I missed my old friends; we shared a lot of fond work memories from over the years. It was refreshing to be reunited with them again.

There was one guest I was eager to approach. When we saw one another, we embraced. I found out only recently that my kindred sister had been a victim of the same supervisor years earlier, but thank God she was in a much better place now. She had spurned his unwanted sexual advances and when she needed a reference he wouldn't give her one. Without a professional recommendation, she had difficulty applying her doctorate degree for work in her chosen field. Instead, she was forced to work in retail for minimum wages.

I finally got around to asking my fellow survivor why she didn't tell me our former boss was crazy, when she knew I was going to work for him. Her answer blew me away. She said it looked like my mind was settled and she didn't want to say anything, if that's what I really wanted. Had it been me, I would have told the new hire to run for her life before it was too late! This manager made the job sound better than it was, and I believed what he told me at the time. I found out that my friend who worked under him was forced into early retirement. My former colleague--the one who had joked about escaping from Alcatraz-- had become management's latest victim after my departure; the abuse took its toll on him as well. When I told this to the woman who was once a victim herself, her response was a chilling one: "Well, it won't be long before he gets another victim."

As soon as she said this I had a revelation: There will be no more victims if I could help it! Had she stood her ground for a cause, just as the goose had, she could have saved the ones coming behind her. It wouldn't have been right had I let someone walk into something that I knew was evil. I would have never forgiven myself had a life been lost because I did not speak up.

Above adversity, I rose with serenity and had the courage to take up a moral cause for the safety of those coming behind me.

SERENITY PRAYER

God, give me grace to accept with serenity

the things that cannot be changed,

Courage to change the things

which should be changed,

and the Wisdom to distinguish

the one from the other.

Living one day at a time,

Enjoying one moment at a time,

Accepting hardship as a pathway to peace,

Taking, as Jesus did,

This sinful world as it is,

Not as I would have it,

Trusting that You will make all things right,

If I surrender to Your will,

So that I may be reasonably happy in this life,

And supremely happy with You forever in the next.

Amen. (Niebuhr, n.d.)

40 *Life, Liberty, and the Pursuit of Depression*

"Job stress can be defined as the harmful physical and emotional responses that occur when the requirements of the job do not match the capabilities, resources, or needs of the worker. Job stress can lead to poor health and even injury."

Centers for Disease Control and Prevention (CDC)

Job stress could also lead to death. I'm puzzled by this definition because it implies that work stress is related to the job's requirements. There was nothing listed in my position description that would have "required" my manager to spiral me into stress-manifested depression. As for what defined a work injury, the Occupational Safety and Health Administration (OSHA) was clear: For an illness or injury to be considered work-related by OSHA, the event or exposure in the work environment had to have either caused or contributed to the resulting condition, or significantly aggravated a pre-existing condition. The irony of my occupational illness was that I worked for a leading health agency.

According to the World Health Organization (WHO), depression is projected to be the second-leading cause of disability worldwide by the year 2020 (Murray & Lopez, 1998). Globally, unipolar depressive disorders were among the top five causes for years of healthy life lost due to disability (YLDs) in 2011 (World Health Organization, 2013) and for the United States, neuropsychiatric disorders were the leading cause of disability in

2010, ahead of cardiovascular and circulatory diseases (National Institute of Mental Health, n.p.).

I should have been able to leave a job the same way I entered it: healthy. What right did a job have to make me suicidal? If the answer was in the data, then it's hard to say. I guess had my supervisor known his actions would paralyze my mind, he might have eased up on the bullying--said the mind that overcame depression, never. What's a worker to do when her manager is an occupational risk?

Wondering how many others had been affected by work-induced mental illness, I searched online for data and statistics. More often than not, I landed at a neatly packaged report bundle of European origin containing facts, charts, and graphs that were easy to interpret. It was during my search that I came across the term *psychological violence*, learning that violence did not necessarily equate to acts of physical harm. Boom!

"Psychological abuse, also referred to as psychological violence, emotional abuse or mental abuse, is a form of abuse characterized by a person subjecting or exposing another to behavior that may result in psychological trauma, including anxiety, chronic depression, or post-traumatic stress disorder. Such abuse is often associated with situations of power imbalance, such as abusive relationships, bullying, and abuse in the workplace." (Wikipedia, 2016) All of the above! It read spot-on, like an excerpt from my work life. In the moment it was both exhilarating and eerie, proof positive I'd been psychologically assaulted on the job.

This definition should be enlarged, laminated, and hung right alongside every company's motto. It should be placed in the lavatories, above the watercoolers, beside the employee time clocks, and converted into table tents and positioned between the salt and pepper shakers on the cafeteria tables. I wondered how different things would have been had the agency referenced this meaning at the onset of my complaints. Or how different it would have been had allegations of psychological harassment carried the same weight as those for sexual harassment. To me, it felt like I'd been intimately violated and harassed.

I have witnessed the swift response on an employee accused of sexual harassment. He was relocated offsite within days. I also saw two colleagues have a tiff, to the point of creating a public spectacle that made others outside the office take notice. One was obviously more aggressive and the other, though less aggressive, argued back while not backing down. The next day, both were terminated. Management made every effort to diffuse the situation and promote harmony before things escalated between the two workers.

Since I had just come from a toxic work environment, I was impressed with how quickly the job intervened to resolve the conflict. Only when it was determined that the arguments appeared volatile enough to become physical, were the employees let go. I believe this was a prime example of respectable leadership, good company ethics, and safe workplace practice.

If asked in a random survey what was the most stressful area of your life, chances are you'd answer "work," for a number of reasons. Suffice it to say that work can play a role on your overall health. Traditionally, more attention has been spent on the physical wellbeing of a worker, and less on a worker's mental health. While the Department of Labor provides adequate resources on workplace violence, what's presented makes no mention of emotional abuse as a component of violence. Yet, in bold capital letters, is the expectation that employees treat each other with dignity and respect for a safe workplace for all (United States Department of Labor, n.p). "Once an employer recognizes that mental health problems are probably the single most important factor responsible for the disability of employees, it makes sense to recognize mental health as a legitimate concern of the organization." (Harnois & Gabriel, 2000)

Given that psychological violence is nothing new and is well known in other countries for its adverse effects in and outside the workplace, it seems feasible this information should have reached the United States by now, even if delivery came by way of a carrier pigeon. Closer to home were two fairly recent cases in Maryland alleging hostile work environments and bullying, as reported in the *Rockville Gazette* (Waibel, 2013) and in the legal recourse sought by Michael Kearns (*Kearns v. Northrop Grumman Systems Corporation*, 2012).

In the first case, former Rockville city employee Charles Baker sued the city, claiming "intolerable" working conditions forced him into early medical retirement after a twenty-nine year career with the city. Mr. Baker alleged that his manager "engaged in unabated and outrageous bullying behavior" that compromised his mental health, and city officials did nothing. In the second case, Michael Kearns filed a lawsuit against his former employer, Northrop Grumman Systems Corporation. Mr. Kearns alleged that he endured retaliation, abusive behavior, and intimidation as a result of an adverse relationship with his supervisor. He claimed these acts were intentional and led to his major depressive disorder and ultimately, his constructive discharge. As in Mr. Baker's the case, Mr. Kearns said that his employer was not helpful.

I could relate to both of these cases. I complained about my manager and became sick when the job failed to step in to resolve our conflict. Unfortunately, my agency never believed there was a conflict to resolve. To them, their leader exercised fair judgment and action over a subordinate who couldn't cut it. Acknowledging that mental wellbeing can be a casualty of work in the United States is half the battle. The other half would be holding managers accountable for psychological abuse and levying hefty fines to employers that did nothing to protect the employee.

I know I wasn't the only employee in America to have been psychologically abused in the workplace. Trying to find statistics for work-induced mental illness cases in the United States produced a migraine within minutes. Mulling over the data felt like I was looking at 4-point font from twenty feet away. So much data was crammed onto one page that it was easy to get lost. That's not to say the information was unavailable; I just had yet to locate it and didn't have a millennium to try. There was data on workplace suicides, even statistics on Blacks and nonfatal occupational injuries and illnesses. However, the data I found didn't suggest what was behind the suicides, or make reference to depression as an occupational illness. Also, federal government cases were nowhere in sight.

This was very disappointing. I did learn that illnesses in the workplace accounted for less than five percent of the nearly three million injury and illness cases in 2014, according to *Employer-Reported Workplace Injury and Illness* (Bureau of Labor Statistics, 2015).

In *Psychology Today*, Canadian leadership coach Ray Williams writes that mental health issues from work are silent tsunamis. I couldn't agree more; I felt that my mental breakdown from work stress was quietly simmering until it boiled over. "Martin Shain, in a recent report for the Mental Health Commission of Canada, titled, *The Road to Psychological Safety: Legal, Scientific and Social Foundations for a national Standard for Psychological Safety,* argues that 'normal' resilient people can be brought to the brink of mental distress and sometimes pushed over the edge by conditions at work." (Williams, 2012)

Stress at Work, a report by the same Canadian commission, implicates managers in exacerbating depression, anxiety, and other common conditions affiliated with workplace mental health (Williams, 2012). Take heed, America: the Mental Health Commission of Canada is telling the truth!

One of the most powerful yet simply worded statements comes from the Vancouver Board of Trade's report *Psychologically Healthy Workplaces: Improving Bottom Line Results and Employee Psychologically Well-Being*: "Protecting psychological well-being is a basic and key element of being a responsible employer." (Williams, 2012) You wouldn't think a report was needed to state the obvious, but if it must be said, then I wish it would be incorporated into a universal work mandate.

Evidence is steady mounting for linking depression and other mental health problems to work. In spite of the evidence, unfortunately, effective interventions for preventing workplace depression remain to be better understood (Centers for Disease Control and Prevention, 2013). If you know the source of the problem (i.e., a supervisor who is making workers depressed), then you can intervene by removing the problem person. In my opinion, that's easy to understand. You'd probably lose one-half of your workforce if you removed the individuals responsible for work-induced mental illness in America. As evident during my ordeal and the statistical fact-finding mission that followed, cases do exist but the data is hard to come by.

Here are some of the key findings from *Physical and Psychological Violence at the Workplace* (Eurofound, 2013):

- Of the diverse types of psychological violence, bullying or general harassment is more prevalent than sexual harassment.

- Research studies indicate psychological violence, particularly bullying, is a social problem of considerable magnitude, with detrimental effects for the health and wellbeing of workers.

- Administrative data shows that an increasing incidence of work-related health problems is due to psychological and psychosocial rather than physical causes.

- Different countries have recognized psychological violence as an occupational risk, equal in importance to other hazards in the work environment.

- Although psychological violence is, by its nature, more cumulative in its impact than physical violence, its negative health effects measured in terms of absenteeism appear to be as detrimental as physical workplace violence.

The Australian Safety and Compensation Council (ASCC) is setting the best example I've seen, with the following bold statements: "The vision of ASCC is Australian workplaces free from injury and disease. Its mission is to lead and coordinate national efforts to prevent workplace death, injury and disease in Australia." (Commonwealth of Australia, 2006)

The late British anti-bullying expert and survivor of workplace bullying, Tim Field, surmised numerous critical points for how bullying in the workplace was accomplished, and it read like my ex-boss's manifesto. It was as if Dr. Field himself had returned from the advocating skies in heaven and walked along beside me, on the job. He described phases of bullying in the workplace that included some of my actual experiences on the job: isolation from colleagues; control beyond work hours; elimination by constructive discharge or medical disability (Tim Field Foundation, 2006).

The United States has a long way to go in addressing psychological abuse in the workplace. To begin with, a new definition of work stress is needed that could go something like this: "Work stress is anything that mentally incapacitates a worker while she is performing her duties." Data must then be collected on work-related mental illness, and timely reports must be made from this data that are not tedious to follow. Address every psychological stressor that has hindered a worker's ability to perform her duties (according to the information in the reports), and track the data to make sure that these occurrences of work-induced depression are declining.

"Mutual respect for the dignity of others at all levels within the workplace is one of the key characteristics of successful organisations. That is why harassment and violence are unacceptable."
Framework agreement on harassment and violence at work
European Social Partners

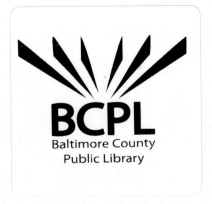

Epilogue: I Have Something to Tell You, America

"No one should have to sacrifice their life for their livelihood, because a nation built on the dignity of work must provide safe working conditions for its people."
Secretary of Labor Thomas E. Perez

Depression is not a cookie-cutter illness; it can look different from person to person, with recovery taking years for some people. Before this book could go to print, a forty-two year-old single mother of three committed suicide in our community after she had lost her job. Her means for ending her life told me she wasn't trying to be saved from death. I could relate to this poor mother who had lost all hope to live. This is why I never gave up on sharing this story, even as obstacles kept getting in the way of completing this book. More women of color are having suicidal thoughts than we may ever know. This single mom was no exception. I was no exception. You are no exception.

What made my depression different was that it got lost in the bureaucracy of a federal agency. I was able to recover from my illness and return to work without the cooperation of the Office of Workers' Compensation Programs (OWCP). This was not how workers' compensation was designed to work. OWCP was designed to help workers during the recovery process, not after.

213

That is, if they helped at all. My claim was still in the appeal phase long after I had resigned from the job that had made me sick.

Alas, vindication! For me, the second time's a charm, instead of the third. Without an attorney or mediator, little ol' me presented a compelling argument about a job that nearly ended my life. Through blood, sweat, and tears, I wrote an appeal--which ultimately resulted in rescinding a denial decision--that has to be the best writing I've ever done. Roughly 145,000 words and 460 pages of relevant correspondences and documents were chronologically arranged, detailing the creation of a twisted work environment over the course of nearly a year. I should earn a Pulitzer Prize nomination for the power of a pen slicing through red tape and jumping over loopholes. I defied the odds and proved that management sank my mental health. Being factual, professional, and respectful, with subdued emotional commentary, won my appeal with OWCP. To God, be the glory!

It's now on record that I sustained personal trauma on the job in the performance of my duties. My workers' compensation claim was accepted more than two years after I was hospitalized, and three years since starting that job. What I had been saying about management from the start was now being corroborated by OWCP. Though elated and grateful for this decision, don't think for one moment that I went frolicking through an enchanted forest to live happily ever after.

Remember when former President Bill Clinton signed into law the IRS (Internal Revenue Service) Overhaul Bill in 1998 that was a lot friendlier to taxpayers, many whom considered the IRS the king of bullies? Well, guess who gets my award for the most incompetent federal agency? Drum roll please…The United States Department of Labor's Office of Workers' Compensation Programs (OWCP), hands down!

Good, timely, accurate, and friendly service would not be OWCP's best traits. Employees I spoke with by phone were curt, sounding almost annoyed I had gotten a phone call through the maze it took to reach a real person. When I first submitted my claim, it took more than four months to receive the first denial, a surprise but no surprise. I then provided more information, but a second denial came three months later. I had been warned that OWCP was tough on psychological injuries. Denials were frequent, acceptances were the Eighth through Tenth Wonders of the World. In the beginning, this is why I believe it was so hard to forge an alliance with lawyers. They must have known my chances for victory were slim to none. The only positive interaction I had with OWCP came with the assistance of my congressman, who got involved after I had complained to him about due process while waiting over a year for the appeal decision following both denials.

OWCP's mission is "to protect the interests of workers who are injured or become ill on the job, their families and their employers by making timely, appropriate, and accurate decisions on claims, providing prompt payment of benefits and helping injured workers return to gainful work as early as is feasible." (US

Department of Labor, n.p.) Their vision statement in part says "OWCP will....earn the trust and respect of those who rely on us for their health and economic well being." (United States Department of Labor, n.p.)

I'm going to leave both of these statements right here because OWCP has not earned my respect at all. My vindication for winning my work-induced depression claim would be even shorter lived as I discovered that back wages would not be automatically granted. OWCP denied my request for wage compensation, citing more evidence was needed. I had to prove I was totally disabled during the dates I had not worked and received no pay. What the what?! As I see it, their mission is to hold your benefits ransom. It was naïve of me to think that OWCP was on the side of the injured worker.

It turned out there were two different decisional processes involved for OWCP claims: one process was for the injury, and the other for compensation. OWCP didn't disclose this compensation addendum until well after my injury claim was accepted. Following OWCP's earlier instructions, I had already submitted the paperwork to receive my compensation from when I was not well enough to work, and I thought my back pay was on its way. I wasn't expecting OWCP to deliver a decision, from a second process I knew nothing about. How could OWCP accept my injury but deny my wages? My God, this was a horrible system!

The medical evidence showed what happened, and my appeal proved how it happened, but now I had to produce further evidence on why I should receive lost pay; and why I had not pursued reasonable accommodations to continue working on the job after my hospitalization.

My suicidal and homicidal ideations should have been the first clues of a tricky puzzle that OWCP didn't seem to want me to solve. OWCP was acting more like a judge rather than as a customer-serving agency. Who knew what an injured mind was capable of, and when? How could I return to the same job and manager that made me sick? That's ridiculous! It wasn't like I was incapacitated beyond ever working again. I had already found a new job elsewhere, no thanks to OWCP. We're talking about a few months' worth of wages, for heaven's sake! If allowed, I would have filed an injury claim against OWCP for the pain and agony of this gut- and mind-wrenching, anxiety-producing process.

If I could put a temporary curse over the entire agency just so it would know what mental illness felt like, I would. Since my mental health emergency, only two events have made me feel as bad as the morning I nearly convinced myself to die. One was finding out that the clinic where I had been in treatment for months would not support my workers' compensation case. The other was when OWCP condescendingly justified why I would not receive any back pay.

I vaguely recalled how, years ago, people had abused personal bankruptcy so much that law-abiding people were adversely affected, such as first-time bankruptcy filers who fell on honest financial hard times. They were assumed to be guilty of abuse before proven innocent. I've never filed for bankruptcy, but would like to think I could without first being prejudged to be financially irresponsible. Then there were the hidden videos capturing people performing strenuous activities when they were supposed to be severely injured and physically limited from compensable work or personal accidents. Was I being punished for my illness by the bureaucracy because workers before me had abused the system? There were always going to be people who tried to take advantage of the system, but those people were actually in the minority. I wasn't one of them.

OWCP was like the old Internal Revenue Service, only a different breed of bully. They didn't snatch your assets away; they withheld them from you, probably banking on you giving up the fight from sheer exhaustion. For every step forward, OWCP found a way to set you back. The enemy who had stolen my mind was now replaced by an agency that had no heart or knowledge of things mental. Why make the honest and deserving suffer?

Fighting for my compensation made me feel like I was a part of a Salem witch trial. If a woman was accused of witchcraft in 17th-century Colonial America, she was given a water test: she was bound and thrown into a body of water to see if she would sink or float, based on an ancient belief that witches floated. If she passed the water test--meaning, the woman sank and drowned--this meant she was innocent. If she floated, she was later executed for being a witch. Innocent or guilty, death was inevitably the outcome for the accused woman.

It was a similar no-win situation when dealing with OWCP. It wasn't enough I suffered a serious psychiatric condition with an open-ended recovery; OWCP made it seem like I would have to die first in order to prove that I had been mentally impacted and entitled to compensation. What a wild-goose chase. If you didn't start off with a mental illness, OWCP might make you develop one.

Well into a new job, I hadn't been treated with psychotherapy and antidepressants for nearly two years. There was no need. I had severed ties with the place that had caused my depression. Unfortunately, I still had unfinished business with OWCP that wouldn't make it a clean break. I began the arduous task of submitting an appeal for the wages I had lost from an old job I was trying very hard to forget. I knew it could take another year for OWCP to accept or deny my claim for lost wages. Even so, life for me was going to move on. I was alive and at peace, intangibles OWCP couldn't deny.

I sent an urgent request for my former psychiatrist to contact me regarding my latest impasse with OWCP. When we spoke by phone more than two years after our last meeting, he remembered me well. Still ever dutiful, he told me to relax while he waited on the delivery of my files that had been in storage; he needed them to write another medical narrative that would either appease or displease the OWCP police.

After OWCP's initial rejection of my injury claim, I began a letter-writing campaign to my local elected officials, describing what had happened to me. I started with the US Office of Special Council and ended with the White House. The legalese and obstacles proved too daunting to continue, fueling why I felt managers--like the one who bullied me--cheated the system of punishment.

Even though my time had long lapsed for filing a complaint with the US Equal Employment Opportunity Commission (EEOC), special consideration should have been made for making a retroactive complaint, since I had an accepted OWCP claim nearly three years post-injury. I had endured retaliatory treatment to the extent where management's "conduct was severe or pervasive enough to create a work environment that a reasonable person would consider intimidating, hostile, or abusive." (US Equal Employment Opportunity Commission, n.p.) If OWCP finally agreed I was made ill by factors relating to employment, then there would be probable grounds that laws had been broken and my civil rights had been violated. Was that reasonable enough? My case would had been a prime example for all agencies that oversee employee rights and welfare to come together to track the employee safety pipeline from occupational illness to prosecution.

Wouldn't it have been just if cases like mine automatically left OWCP's desk and landed on the desk of the Department of Justice, resulting in manager firings at least and jail terms at best? You can't take mean managers, haul them off into some kind of anti-bullying training, and then return them to duty with an expectation that things will change for a happier workplace. Once a menace, always a menace. My bully was driven by power and control. Remove his authority to supervise, cut off his funding until he completes mandated therapy, and keep him on probation so there is always a watchful eye. Fine these managers in the five figures, or ten percent of compensatory damages--whichever is higher--before having his picture posted on the Federal Bureau of Investigation's Managers Least Wanted list. Use any fines collected to bully-proof the workplace moving forward.

Less than a year after my unplanned institutionalization, someone from the former job broke a cardinal workplace rule: he made a physical connection with the ex-boss, only I wished he had connected a lot harder and injured more than management's self-importance. If you knew this worker--whose soul was so gentle and peaceful--you'd know that would have been like Martin Luther King, Jr. not practicing what he preached. Once a bully backs you into a corner with no escape, there's no telling how you'd react. My reaction was internal: I suffered emotional damage. For my good friend who lashed out against management with a different response, I was just sorry his actions cost him his job.

Now that another employee was forced off the job under alarming circumstances, inquiring minds are still asking what has become of this unhinged manager. The answer remains the same: nothing. He is still on the job, poisoning the reputation of the agency with his amoral venom.

My case is protected under the Privacy Act; therefore, OWCP will not share the particulars of the report with anyone without regard for my confidentiality. So how will the agency know what infractions caused my occupational illness, and how will they respond to what management has done? I could share the contents of the report with the agency should I choose; however, the agency may do more for his rights than they ever did for mine, based on my experience with them. If I've calculated correctly, the agency may have to reimburse my insurance carrier--for over a year's worth of mental health treatment, and the equivalent of that large settlement that may have been granted to me, had I been able to seek a judgment award in time. This may hit home harder than any report could. It's not the justice I'd prefer, but it's better than nothing.

There was a newsworthy article alleging that there were Animal Welfare Act violations at Johns Hopkins University in Baltimore, due to research primates being so stressed out from mistreatment. The United States Department of Agriculture (USDA) issued a stern warning to Hopkins; an animal rights group demanded a stiff fine (Titus, 2016). If there is compassion and oversight for lab animals, then I'd like to think that I, and others, matter as much as any other primate and have a right to ethical treatment in the workplace. All it will take is for that one employee who is pushed too far, for you to extrapolate what will next happen to management.

I was a few years into working at my wonderful, new job when I suffered a significant sprain that affected my ability to perform my duties. What were the chances I'd be injured at work, a second time? I couldn't believe my misfortune. I would have done anything to avoid going through workers' compensation, again. The previous claims process--which still hadn't been settled after more than three years--was not kind to me to all.

I was not prepared for what happened next: my case was accepted immediately after I had filed the claim. I received a prescription card to cover any medications related to my injury. And my medical bills went directly to workers' compensation to eliminate my out of pocket expenses. I was in shock; this had to be a dream. The representative assigned to my case was cordial, reachable, and helpful--everything the OWCP workers that I had encountered were not. This time, the workers' compensation process was efficient and superb! I would have never believed that it helped the injured employee like it was supposed to by "addressing the needs of the injured worker in a timely and caring manner." This insurance carrier for workers' compensation was true to its motto.

It didn't take mounds of paperwork and years to prove I had been injured on the job, as was the case for OWCP. Rather, all it took was a brief statement from the job, and a workers' compensation representative phoning my doctor. I didn't have to do much at all, except get treated and get well. The job fully supported my recovery, and allowed me to adjust to a modified work schedule while I was being treated. My supervisor made me feel important, even if I wasn't at full strength. Aside from getting hurt, I'd say this was a pleasant process.

The US Department of Labor's Office of Workers' Compensation Programs--with a federal staff of over 1,700 and an annual operating budget of $345,000,000--was just embarrassed by the workers' compensation insurance for a small, private sector company. The hapless way OWCP managed my case was a disservice to the injured federal worker; it did not depict the best that a government agency had to offer. I would love to see the data for how many OWCP employees and labor hours were used on my case, alone. How much had my case cost the government? The world may never know, America. I wouldn't be surprised if my back wages were less than what it cost for OWCP to work on my still pending case. What a sham, and a shame!

"The victim who is able to articulate the situation of the victim has ceased to be a victim: he or she has become a threat."
James Baldwin

Notes

Bureau of Labor Statistics. (2015). *Employer-Reported Workplace Injury and Illness Summary*. Retrieved 18 February, 2016, from http://www.bls.gov/news.release/osh.nr0.htm

Centers for Disease Control and Prevention. (2013). *Depression*. Retrieved 18 February, 2016, from http://www.cdc.gov/workplacehealthpromotion/implementation/topics/depression.html

Commonwealth of Australia. (2006). WORK-RELATED MENTAL DISORDERS IN AUSTRALIA. Retrieved 21 February, 2016, from http://www.safeworkaustralia.gov.au/sites/SWA/about/Publications/Documents/416/Workrelated_Mental_Disorders_Australia.pdf

Eurofound (2013), *Physical and psychological violence at the workplace*, Publications Office of the European Union, Luxembourg.

Harnois, G., & Gabriel, P. (2000). *Mental health and work: Impact, issues and good practices*. Geneva: World Health Organization.

Lopez, A. D., & Murray, C. C. (1998). The global burden of disease, 1990–2020. *Nature Medicine Nat Med*, 4(11), 1241-1243.

Michael Kearns v. Northrop Grumman Systems Corporation (United States District Court for the District of Maryland 2012), (Online). United States Government Printing Office. Retrieved 18 February, 2016, from https://www.gpo.gov/fdsys/pkg/USCOURTS-mdd-1_11-cv-01736/pdf/USCOURTS-mdd-1_11-cv-01736-0.pdf

National Institute of Mental Health. (n.p.). *US Leading Categories of Diseases/Disorders*. Retrieved 23 February, 2016, from https://www.nimh.nih.gov/health/statistics/disability/us-leading-categories-of-diseases-disorders.shtml

Niebuhr, R. (n.p.). Serenity Prayer. Retrieved 17 February, 2016, from
http://en.wikipedia.org/wiki/Serenity_Prayer

Ogden, J., Sr. (2013). *Faith or Fear*. Retrieved February 17, 2016, from
https://www.facebook.com/cmawonbyonechapter.cma/posts/41343
5452081954

Tim Field Foundation. (2006). *What is Workplace Bullying?*
Retrieved 18 February, 2016, from
http://bullyonline.org/index.php/bullying/19-what-is-workplace-bullying

Titus, R. (2016, March 18). JHU hit with 'official warning' from
USDA for mistreatment of monkeys. *WBFF Fox45 News*.
Retrieved from http://foxbaltimore.com/news/local/john-hopkins-hit-with-official-warning-from-udsa-for-mistreatment-of-monkeys

Tully, M. B. (2014). *Government Pays the Price for Making Fed
Employees Depressed*. Retrieved February 19, 2016, from
http://www.fedsmith.com/2014/05/20/government-pays-the-price-for-making-fed-employees-depressed/

United States Department of Labor. (n.p.). *DOL Workplace
Violence Program*. Retrieved 18 February, 2016, from
http://www.dol.gov/oasam/hrc/policies/dol-workplace-violence-program.htm

United States Department of Labor. (n.p.). *US Department of
Labor - Office of Workers' Compensation Programs (OWCP) -
Mission, Vision, Goals*. Retrieved February 19, 2016, from
http://www.dol.gov/owcp/owcpmisvisgols.htm

US Equal Employment Opportunity Commission. (n.p.). *Harassment.* Retrieved 20 February, 2016, from http://www.eeoc.gov/laws/types/harassment.cfm

Waibel, E. (2013, September 18). Former Rockville city employee sues for 'intolerable' work conditions. *Gazette Rockville.* Retrieved from https://issuu.com/thegazette/docs/rockvillegaz_091813

Wikipedia.org. (2016). *Psychological abuse.* Retrieved 17 February, 2016, from https://en.wikipedia.org/wiki/Psychological_abuse

Williams, R. (2012). *The Silent Tsunami: Mental Health in the Workplace.* Retrieved 18 February, 2016, from https://www.psychologytoday.com/blog/wired-success/201209/the-silent-tsunami-mental-health-in-the-workplace

World Health Organization. (2013). *WHO methods and data sources for global burden of disease estimates 2000-2011.* Retrieved 23 February, 2016, from http://www.who.int/healthinfo/statistics/GlobalDALYmethods_2000_2011.pdf?ua=1

Photo Credits

Front/Back Cover
Emerson, T. (Photographer). (n.d.). Reflected Riparian Tree and
Canadian Geese in Golden Sunset. [Digital Image]. Retrieved
from
http://image.shutterstock.com/display_pic_with_logo/92656/92656
,1203707476,11/stock-photo-reflected-riparian-tree-and-canadian-
geese-in-golden-sunset-9684568.jpg

Part I
Lone Wolf Photography (Photographer). (n.d.). Canadian Goose
Flying Against a Sunset in Maryland. [Digital Image]. Retrieved
from
http://image.shutterstock.com/display_pic_with_logo/551986/5519
86,1303938626,1/stock-photo-canadian-goose-flying-against-a-
sunset-in-maryland-76094158.jpg

Part II
Murray, I. (Photographer). (n.d.). Bald Eagle with Goose Dinner.
[Digital image]. Retrieved from
https://www.flickr.com/photos/wallaceriver/8330367563

Part III
Burgener, R. (Photographer). (2014). Meet Bert and Ernie. [Digital
image]. Retrieved from
http://www.about.lovecanadageese.com/bertandernie.html

Part IV
Diaz, J. (Photographer). (2011). Canada Goose Taking Off.
[Digital image]. Retrieved from
https://www.flickr.com/photos/koolpix_nature/5899661376/

Part V
Shake, M. (Photographer). (n.d.). Photo of Canadian Geese Flying in Formation. Taken On the Scenic Maumee River in Northwest Ohio. [Digital image]. Retrieved from http://image.shutterstock.com/display_pic_with_logo/493/1829598 05/stock-photo-photo-of-canadian-geese-flying-in-formation-taken-on-the-scenic-maumee-river-in-northwest-ohio-182959805.jpg

Back Cover Inset
Sheradon, A. (Photographer). (2015). Taking Off. [Digital Image]. Retrieved from https://www.flickr.com/photos/viv3rai/17357969091/in/photostream/

Appendix
Burgener, R. (Photographer). (2016) Used by permission.

Related Resources

Bureau of Labor Statistics. (2013). *Workplace Homicides.* Retrieved 18 February, 2016, from http://www.bls.gov/iif/workplace_homicides_20130917.htm

Centers for Disease Control and Prevention. (2009). *WORK ORGANIZATION AND STRESS-RELATED DISORDERS.* Retrieved 20 February, 2016, from http://www.cdc.gov/niosh/programs/workorg/

Centers for Disease Control and Prevention. (2013). *STRESS AT WORK.* Retrieved 20 February, 2016, from http://www.cdc.gov/niosh/topics/stress/

Centers for Disease Control and Prevention. (2015). *The Changing Employment Relationship and Its Impact on Worker Well-Being.* Retrieved 20 February, 2016, from http://www.cdc.gov/niosh/enews/enewsV12N12.html

Crosby, A. E. & Molock, S.D. (2006). Introduction: Suicidal Behaviors in the African American Community. *Journal of Black Psychology, 32*(3), 253-261.

Krause, B. (2011). *"Fear-Based" PTSD Criteria Explained.* Retrieved April 25, 2016, from http://militaryadvantage.military.com/2011/06/fear-based-ptsd-criteria-explained/

Minkove, J.F. (2015). *Combining Genes, Epigenetics and Stress Responses to Study Suicide and PTSD.* Retrieved April 5, 2016, from http://www.hopkinsmedicine.org/news/articles/combining-genes-epigenetics-and-stress-responses-to-study-suicide-and-ptsd

Murray, C. J., & Lopez, A. D. (1996). *The global burden of disease; summary.* Geneva: World Health Organization.

Occupational Safety & Health Administration. (n.p.). *Federal Injury and Illness Statistics for Fiscal Year 2014*. Retrieved 20 February, 2016, from https://www.osha.gov/dep/fap/statistics/fedrprgrms_stats14_final.html

Oppermman, S. (2008). *Workplace Bullying: Psychological Violence?* Retrieved February 20, 2016, from http://www.fedsmith.com/2008/12/03/workplace-bullying-psychological-violence/

Szymendera, Scott D. (2016). *The Federal Employees' Compensation Act (FECA): Workers' Compensation for Federal Employees* (CRS Report No. R42107). Retrieved from Congressional Research Service. https://www.fas.org/sgp/crs/misc/R42107.pdf

World Health Organization. (c2016). *Estimates for 2000–2012 DISEASE BURDEN*. Retrieved 24 February 2016, from http://www.who.int/healthinfo/global_burden_disease/estimates/en/index2.html

Woo, J., & Postolache, T. T. (2008). The impact of work environment on mood disorders and suicide: Evidence and implications. *International Journal on Disability and Human Development, 7*(2), 185-200.

Zanolli, N. (2002). *When Conflict In The Workplace Escalates To Emotional Abuse*. Retrieved February 20, 2016, from http://www.mediate.com/articles/davenport.cfm

Acknowledgements

I am indebted to a flock of supporters whose unwavering love and care brought me back from the brink of death. They stayed by my side from the onset, and refused to leave me until my wounds had healed. Thank you Gerald, Ricky, Sheila, Althea, Antoinette, Felecia, Shelia, Patricia, Lena, Adranna, Krystle, and Wilbert! To the courageous employees who backed me with supporting statements that helped seal a legal victory, thank you!

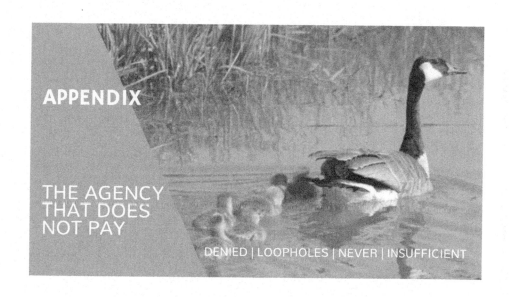

APPENDIX

THE AGENCY
THAT DOES
NOT PAY

DENIED | LOOPHOLES | NEVER | INSUFFICIENT

The Accidental Injured Worker

The pitfalls of being an accidental, mentally impaired worker are knowing that your impairment was an intentional accident; knowing that you have to pass through an impenetrable vault known as the Office of Workers' Compensation Programs (OWCP); and feeling as if you're the derelict of the work force. In corresponding with OWCP regarding my mental illness, I can't tell you if some of their written responses to my claims were automated, but I can tell you that they lacked empathy. I often wondered if I was communicating with a human or a robot.

I knew I had a strong case, but could have never predicted how long and strong a fight OWCP would put me through to make them believe that my mental illness was acquired from the job. It was a tremendous battle but thankfully, I had a few things working for me:

- I was driven by morals and the thoughts of saving other sufferers.
- My motive was not vengeance against the perpetrator, but change for a safer workplace.
- I had found work and retained income while fighting with OWCP.

- My psychiatrist did what he was required to do ethically, and rendered his honest medical opinion that corroborated my account of events.
- I was able to maneuver through the difficult OWCP process without a labor attorney.
- I was moderately organized and reasonably articulate when writing my defense against the denials.
- I was patient enough to stay the course, in spite of OWCP's procrastination and resistance.
- I enlisted the help of my local congressman.
- I had very good health insurance before I was injured on the job; this sustained me for several months while I was on medical leave.
- I had saved a long email trail, with incriminating evidence against management. I was able to use this successfully in my claim.

When I thought about all the people suffering from work-induced mental illness who did not have the advantages I had, it's no wonder many claims were dropped, if reported at all. What we all have in common, I think, is our inability to pay a good lawyer. But should it have taken suicidal thoughts, an emergency hospitalization, and months under a psychiatrist to prove mental illness from work? What would happen if all of the workers who became mentally ill from work, but were unable to pass OWCP's rigid requirements for compensation, filed a class action lawsuit?

If a physician, who was not a psychiatrist, prescribed antidepressants and declared that a worker had no mental health history prior to starting a new job, then shouldn't that be enough to pass the mental detector test for claiming psychological impairment to even a slight degree? If it was that simple, I imagine OWCP would go bankrupt. Surely the diagnosis should be left to a psychiatrist.

Despite two different psychiatrists rendering post-traumatic stress disorder, OWCP said there was no evidence my PTSD diagnosis was linked to factors of my employment. My psychiatrist and I were irate. To this day, there are certain triggers that set my mental health on edge. Someone at first glance who resembles my ex-boss; the many businesses and roads that share his last name that I've noticed since coming away from that experience; and specific phrases and words he used in my daily beratings. OWCP accepted only my major depressive disorder, which had many of the same symptoms as PTSD. The only way to have post-trauma is to have experienced trauma beforehand. An accepted PTSD condition could probably have me on claim support for life, in my conspiracy thinking, to explain why OWCP wouldn't accept this diagnosis that had been thrice confirmed by my psychiatrists--magna cum laude graduates, national medical honor society members, board certified practicing psychiatrists with over 70 years of experience, collectively. When did OWCP become the leading authority on PTSD?

It's odd that my disability was questioned the moment I exhausted my paid leave and switched over to unpaid status, for which OWCP was supposed to jump in and assist with my "economic well being." As long as I was paying for being disabled, things were cool. But when my pay ran out, OWCP demanded proof that I was disabled during the nonpaid portion. What kind of system would pay for your medical expenses related to your work injury, refund the health care insurance provider for their portion of medical services rendered for the work injury, but not pay your lost wages for a few months from the same injury? Case in point: I was reimbursed by OWCP for the cost of the additional medical documentation I needed to validate my disability for compensation, since my medical expenses (e.g., office visits, phone consultations, prescribed medications, etc.) had been accepted and approved for my claim. Again, OWCP paid for the medical report required to prove my disability.

I want to pick up where I left off in the epilogue, with the mission and vision of OWCP. OWCP was a hurry-up-and-wait agency: I was timely with my claims, but OWCP was untimely with their decisions. The Office of Workers' Compensation Programs failed miserably in protecting my interests. My claim could have dragged on for many more years, had I not asked my congressman to investigate what was taking OWCP so long on the injury appeal. If I had to adhere to thirty-day deadlines for submissions, why didn't OWCP have to do so as well when rendering decisions? I had been extremely meticulous when submitting my medical reimbursement claims; they looked like well-organized, professional reports that were complete with charts, graphs, and tables. However, OWCP would return my claims because information was allegedly missing or invalid, while at the same time informing me I had missed my opportunity for reimbursements by not filing within the allotted amount of time. Lies! Nothing was missing, invalid, or expired. All of the errors for processing my claims came from within OWCP.

I filed reimbursement claims for my injury within weeks of the acceptance decision, but it was evident someone had yet to tell the workers of OWCP that my case was approved. It was unbelievable how much time and energy were wasted trying to get what I had been cleared to receive. OWCP was notorious for telling me to re-submit my claims all over again--claims that were never lost to begin with, just entangled in their negligence.

If this wasn't baffling enough, OWCP wanted evidence that I had requested reasonable accommodations within any restrictions from my employer. If you've been following the timeline, then how could I relay such a request to an employer I hadn't worked for in two years? Remember, my case was retroactive. OWCP didn't accept my major depressive disorder diagnosis until after I'd left the agency. I couldn't do what OWCP asked, unless I traveled back into the past in a time machine. In addition, my psychiatrist made it clear in the medical narrative that I was unable to return to the job with the manager in question due to my medical diagnoses. Now I'm convinced I was dealing with robots.

Thank God this wasn't my fight, but the Lord's. This is what I had to remind myself of whenever I wanted to imagine sending a drone to level an empty OWCP headquarters. No lives harmed, just the disintegration of flawed policies and dated practices. OWCP needed to start afresh from the ground up.

Their vision "to be an innovative leader in the delivery of benefits" failed as bad as their mission when it came to my case. Service was horrible when I first filed my claim, and it was still horrible years later, with nothing changing for the better over the progression of time. In theory, my reimbursement claims were supposed to be submitted within a year after the date in which service was provided or the date that my case was first accepted, even if the acceptance came more than a year post-injury. The reality was that OWCP's computer system couldn't tell time beyond a year, defaulting to denying every claim submission I sent because the claims were dated after the one-year time limit. OWCP's "robots" were dumb. Not a very innovating infrastructure, if you asked me. The agency also failed every goal they set for delivering high quality service. For me, the service I received was of the lowest quality.

The Office of Workers' Compensation Programs must honor its mission, vision, and goals if it wants to be known for delivering premium care to injured workers. Unfortunately, OWCP has long been reputed as the agency that does not care. What is the point of having insurance if it won't pay when you're hurt? The road this accidental mentally impaired worker traveled to an accepted OWCP medical claim was as bumpy a ride as you'll ever get, and as winding and crooked as San Francisco's Lombard Street. My mind got away from me once when it was raped by a bully in the workplace. My mission is to never let this happen to me again, with a vision of keeping it from happening to you too, for a workplace that is free of bullying.

Final Thoughts

Not all places of employment are health risks. Today's workplaces are evolving into great places to work. Cafeterias have been revamped to provide healthier choices for employee wellness. Companies are helping the environment by reducing waste and recycling more. Employers recognize that the quality of life beyond work influences a worker's productivity at work. Jobs are incorporating fitness and fun activities into the bustle of a workday to sustain the morale of its workers. Some employees are given paid time-off to volunteer for causes that are important to them. These are the kinds of workplaces that value and engage employees. Workers are happy, and employers have a high retention rate.

Even smoking at work isn't what it used to be. You always knew when an employee returned from a smoke break: the worker reeked of smoke long after the break had ended. Businesses are transitioning to tobacco-free workplaces with the health of the employee in mind. Ashtrays in the workplace have been replaced with smoking igloos on the grounds of the workplace, until finally workplaces developed non-smoking policies, where you couldn't smoke inside or outside the work site, period. Treat bullying like a smoking addiction, and stop it cold in its tracks without accommodating it. Otherwise, its odor will linger and continue to offend and distress the rest of the workplace.

About the Author

Lisa G. Eley graduated from Baltimore's Western High School, the oldest public all-girls high school remaining in the U.S., and she holds a biology degree from Towson University. Passionate about many causes, Lisa devotes her life to serving the needs of the community and is a strong advocate for narrowing the academic achievement gap. She is the author of *Packet of Opportunities for College Bound Students*, a complimentary scholarship resources guide listing hundreds of scholarships and internship opportunities specific for underserved populations. Lisa is a member of Zeta Phi Beta Sorority, Inc. and is a contributing author to the anthologies *Keeping it Finer: What it Means to be a Finer Woman in the 21st Century* (Crystal Stairs, Inc., 2015) and *Scholarship: Wisdom and Intellect for the 21st Century* (Crystal Stairs, Inc., 2016).

CPSIA information can be obtained
at www.ICGtesting.com
Printed in the USA
LVOW13s2125220217
525103LV00016B/771/P